THE 17 DAY

KICK-START DIET

THE 17 DAY
KICK-START DIET

A DOCTOR'S PLAN FOR DROPPING POUNDS, TOXINS, AND BAD HABITS

MIKE MORENO, MD

ATRIA BOOKS

NEW YORK   LONDON   TORONTO   SYDNEY   NEW DELHI

ATRIA
BOOKS

An Imprint of Simon & Schuster, Inc.
1230 Avenue of the Americas
New York, NY 10020

First Atria Books hardcover edition December 2021

ATRIA BOOKS and colophon are trademarks of Simon & Schuster, Inc.

For information about special discounts for bulk purchases, please contact Simon & Schuster Special Sales at 1-866-506-1949 or business@simonandschuster.com.

The Simon & Schuster Speakers Bureau can bring authors to your live event. For more information or to book an event, contact the Simon & Schuster Speakers Bureau at 1-866-248-3049 or visit our website at www.simonspeakers.com.

Interior design by Jill Putorti

Manufactured in the United States of America

1 3 5 7 9 10 8 6 4 2

Library of Congress Cataloging-in-Publication Data has been applied for.

ISBN 978-1-9821-6062-3
ISBN 978-1-9821-6064-7 (ebook)

MEDICAL DISCLAIMER

This book is dedicated to my family and friends who have supported me in my life efforts and dreams, to my sister and my dear mother, and to my girlfriend who continuously supports me and reminds me to believe in myself. It is so exhilarating to see this project come to completion. I hope everyone who picks up this book enjoys what they read. I humbly and hopefully request that anyone who reads this tries to use it as a template and guide for their own life. My hope is that it serves as an opportunity to reflect on the things in your life that have molded you into who you are today. I truly believe this is a fantastic plan for creating a better body, inside and out.

CONTENTS

THE 17 DAY
KICK-START DIET

INTRODUCTION

Hello there! It's been a while. In fact, it's been over a decade since you and I first talked about how you could lose weight rapidly in *The 17 Day Diet*. I'm sure a lot has happened in your life since then, and a lot has certainly happened in mine. In fact, I've lived through some of my highest highs and many of my lowest lows in these last ten years.

But here we are, you and I, still chugging along on this journey called life. We decide our destination and how we're going to get there, and our bodies are really just along for the ride. As a doctor, I'm constantly amazed at what the body is capable of, especially when we give it what it needs. I have witnessed patients make incredible transformations, ones in which their bodies go from busted up and broken down to bouncing with life and brimming with energy. If we want our bodies to carry us through life's adventures, we've got to take care of them. But we don't do that with an "all or nothing" mentality, where we deprive ourselves of things we enjoy. What I've come to understand, both in my own life and through those of thousands of patients, is that our bodies respond best to a simple philosophy: more of the good, less of the bad.

I know, that sounds so simple. And that's because it is. I've just seen so many people swing on that pendulum between the "starvation diet" and the "all-you-can-eat buffet" mentality, and neither extreme ever leads to optimal health. But if we can strive to live each day choosing more of the good and less of the bad, then we can know what it is to live a fulfilling, healthy life. And I'm referring not only to good or bad food. I'm referring to the multitude of lifestyle choices that affect us.

Here's the deal: we can never anticipate what life is going to dish up. Too many factors are outside of our control. But we *can* choose to approach each day as a fresh start. I know this from firsthand experience. In 2011, I was forty-four years old and a lifelong bachelor. I had pretty much decided I was never going to get married. And then fate intervened and I met the woman who would become my wife. We bought a beautiful home and built a life with our two cats and dog. I was the happiest I had ever been. Everything just felt so stable, so secure, and as a result, I started packing on the pounds. Of course, I didn't realize it when it was happening (do we ever?), but when we were staying at a hotel one Thanksgiving, I hopped on the scale just to see, and sure enough, I had gained 35 pounds. Thirty-five! I had gone from the 175-pound weight I'd been for as long as I could remember all the way up to 210 pounds. Sure, I'd been swimming five days a week just like always, but I had also been eating anything I wanted, and plenty of it. I had become what I've often referred to as "fit fat." I'd forgotten the 90/10 rule that I tell all my patients—weight management is 90 percent food intake and 10 percent exercise.

A Picture Is Worth A Thousand Words

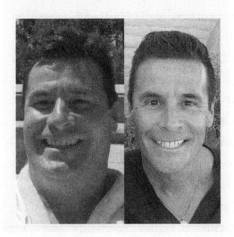

I snapped a photo of the reading on the scale and sent it to my brother with the caption, "Uh-oh!" He couldn't believe it either. "Whose weight is that?" he asked. "Mine!" I replied. We had a good laugh, and I joked that I better read my own book again. But truth be told, I didn't really care. I was married, I was happy, and, yeah, I was a little overweight. So what?

When my wife and I decided to start a family, our state of bliss was suddenly disrupted. We experienced fertility issues. Both she and I got checked out, and it appeared that everything was in working order, but even so, she lost several pregnancies. I can't even explain how painful it was watching her go through miscarriages over and over. After some time, we made the mutual decision that we weren't meant to have kids. And we were totally okay with it. Or so I thought.

I'll never know the real reason why, but one morning when I woke up, she looked me in the eye and said the words that shattered my world: "This isn't working for me." I was devastated. She had no interest in discussing it or trying to save the marriage; she was done. Overnight, I went from being this happy guy with a big house, a great job, and an amazing wife, to being an empty shell of myself. If it wasn't for my friends, I'm not sure how I would have made it through that time in my life. I never missed a day of work, though there were many times I'd be crying alone in my office between patients. As soon as the weekend arrived, I'd drive the two hours up to Los Angeles from San Diego so I could be out of that house where we'd built a life together. I just couldn't bear to be in that space—it hurt too much.

For nine months, I was numb. To ease the pain in those lonely hours after work, I drank. I drank *a lot*. And I smoked cigars. I ate terribly. I'm the kind of person who can't eat much when I'm under stress, so I started losing weight, but for all the wrong reasons. I knew logically that I should make the stress of the situation work for me, but I just didn't have it in me. My best friend of forty-five years had been through something similar, and he told me how it was going to play out. He said, "You're going to feel like shit for a while. You'll ask a bunch of questions, but you'll never get answers, and even if you do, you won't know if they

are accurate. You'll drink a lot, and you'll do other self-destructive behaviors. But eventually, you'll stop. You'll slowly begin to feel yourself
returning. And you *will* be okay." I trusted him, but it was hard to believe
when I was in the thick of those emotions.

Finally, in February of 2018, about eighteen months after the divorce,
I decided to put the house up for sale. I rented a condo downtown close
to some friends of mine, and two days after I moved in, I felt like I had
been reborn. My buddy had been right; I was starting to return to myself. It was like I was coming out of a thick fog, and the sunlight was
breaking through.

And then my nephew called and said, "I think your sister is sick."

Now, I'll pause here and share with you that I come from a big family, and we are very tight-knit. I have six siblings; I'm the youngest. Less
than a year prior, Stephanie, my sister (we called her Stevie for short),
had lost her husband to pulmonary fibrosis, an idiopathic lung disease
that is just downright nasty. They'd been married for fifty-five years, so
it was very rough on her. She had been completely miserable since he
had died.

I asked what was going on, and my nephew said she'd gone to the
doctor because she was yellow, which was a sign that she was jaun-
diced, and they'd discovered a mass. I went into doctor mode immediately and told him, "Listen, I hate to tell you this, but it's probably
cancer. And it's probably a bad cancer. But let's get some tests done and
go from there."

A few hours later, I was still trying to wrap my head around the fact
that my sister was so sick and it felt so sudden, and then my phone
rang again. It was my other sister, Lynn. "Mike, Mom had a big stroke,"
she said. The news hit me square in the chest. "What?! Are you kidding
me?" Was it really possible that both my sister and my mom had fallen
seriously ill . . . *on the same day*? It just didn't make sense. My mind was
reeling.

It turned out my mom had a massive hemorrhage in her brain, and
it was a hospice situation. And my sister's diagnosis? Pancreatic cancer.
My brother stayed with her for a few days while they did some testing,

and we decided not to tell her that Mom was in hospice with a serious brain bleed. And my mom was too out of it to comprehend much of anything, so I didn't tell her about my sister's diagnosis. By the Sunday of that week, they determined my sister would also go on hospice.

My brother called me on the following Thursday when I'd just gotten out of work and said, "You probably need to come up here pretty soon." This was just ten days after the initial finding. They had tried to do a procedure, but her pressure dropped, her heart rate plummeted, and they had to put her on pressors. She was stable, but we agreed I'd fly up there in the morning.

I was on the airplane, shortly before takeoff, when my cell phone rang. I went to answer it, but the flight attendant said I had to turn off my phone. Being the rule follower that I am, I ignored the call and figured I could wait; it was just a two-hour flight. I called my brother back as soon as I got off the plane. "Mike, I tried calling you. She died this morning." I had so wanted to see her to say goodbye, but it had just all happened so fast.

My mom remained in hospice until the end of that year. She didn't know who we were, and from the moment she had the stroke, she never returned to the woman we'd known our entire lives. She was alive, but she wasn't living, if you know what I mean. In December of 2018, one of my sisters called me and said Mom didn't look good and I should come up. I drove up on a Friday, and right as I was parking my car in the lot outside, she called again and told me that Mom was gone. I'd missed my chance to say goodbye . . . again. But I had spent a lot of time with her over those months. And I was grateful that my mom had passed peacefully, having never realized that my sister had preceded her in death.

We take things for granted sometimes, and then when trauma hits, our resiliency gets tested. I had always been my mom's favorite, the baby of the family, and losing her was really difficult. She taught me so much, and to this day, her voice is almost constantly in my head. (And it will soon be in yours, too, as I'll be sharing some of her beautiful life wisdom with you in these pages.) It just doesn't matter at what age we lose a parent—it's always hard. I understood conceptually that life must go on, of course, but I was a mess inside.

My divorce had felt very much like a death to me, but then to be so quickly followed by the passing of my sister and my mom, well, it was a lot to handle. Luckily, I haven't had to go through it all alone. I have the most amazing friends, a couple of whom you'll hear about throughout this book. I have a girlfriend who has been by my side for the last three years as well, and she has been hugely supportive and compassionate. Really, she's one of the most thoughtful humans I know. Always calm and methodical in her thinking, she pays exceptional attention to detail. I can't adequately articulate all that she's done for me over the years. I have a lot to learn from her, that's for sure.

I also have a fantastic therapist. That's right, this doctor is in therapy. I often share that with my patients, too, because I think too many folks wrongly believe that asking for help is a sign of weakness, when really it's quite the opposite. It's a sign of strength and self-awareness. Therapy is where I can process what's going on in my life, and where I can connect the dots to my past, even when it's painful to do so. The truth is, if we don't do that, the past has a funny way of showing up. Maybe you've noticed that in your own life. Dealing with our emotions, working through our experiences, it's all part of our overall picture of health and well-being. And honestly, it's because of the tools I've learned in therapy that my ex-wife and I have, over time, become friends. We talk to each other about our lives, and we've both come to realize that even when relationships don't work out, friendships can still blossom.

I'm opening up this book by sharing some of my personal story with you because I want you to begin to think about your *own* story. We all have one. And when we take the time to really connect with our life story, we are able to give ourselves a little more grace. We are able to cut ourselves some slack and realize that life, at times, can be incredibly demanding. It can be rocky. Our job is to find a way to prioritize our health along the way, without beating ourselves up about it. It is to know who we are and what works for us, and not to put unrealistic expectations on ourselves. We are often our own worst critics, am I right? But when we look at our lives and consider all the ups and downs, peaks and valleys, we can see that we are worthy and deserving of respect and care. I'm not saying our experiences are excuses, but rather incredible feats we have accomplished. And just imagine how much more we can rise to whatever occasion life dishes up if we are coming into it with a solid foundation of health. That's why I want you to think about your story, to connect with it in new ways, and to take part in writing your own next chapter.

Sometimes our health plays a starring role in our life story. Like so many of my patients and the wonderful folks in my online and social media communities, I'm on my own unique health journey at the moment. It all started about four years ago when I went to the bathroom (yes, I'm going there with you), and I peed blood. Alarming, I know. I immediately went to see my urologist and we started a battery of tests. Including a urinary scope. Ouch. They found a lot of inflammation, and I had to do a couple rounds of antibiotics. The problem seemed to resolve after that.

That is, until recently, when I started experiencing excruciating pain around my pubic bone and my lower back. I lost about ten pounds in a month, and I was having to lie down flat on my back in my office between patients. When I was driving, I had to pull the lap belt off my lap. Yeah, it wasn't good. And then I wasn't really able to urinate except for just dribbles. All of my doctor instincts were screaming at me to take action.

One CT scan, an ultrasound, and another urinary scope later, we learned that, once again, there was a ton of inflammation but, thank goodness, no signs of cancer. It was time for more antibiotics, anti-inflammatory medications, and absolutely no caffeine or alcohol. There was some improvement, but not enough. And my back pain was getting worse. I went in for an MRI.

The radiologist called with my results, and led with the good news. Nothing life-threatening. But then he asked, "Do you know about your hips?" Um, I have hips, yes, I do know that. I wondered what he meant. "You have avascular necrosis in both of your hips," he continued. What?! How could that be? Avascular necrosis, which essentially means a loss of blood supply to the bone, was usually caused by many years of smoking, or some kind of physical trauma to the region. But in my case, it was idiopathic, meaning no specific cause. There's no cure, and no reversing the disease progression. It sort of is what it is.

It was a shocking diagnosis, to say the least. I'm fifty-two years old, very active, and I lead a healthy, busy, and rewarding life. This condition is going to require some pretty heavy lifestyle changes. I'll never run, jog, or climb stairs for exercise again, but I'm a swimmer, and that's the perfect exercise for me. At some point in the future, I will need to have surgery on my hips, but for now I'm choosing to focus on how grateful I am that it wasn't something worse.

I know there are millions of people out there who are living with chronic pain. There are a multitude of causes for that pain, from conditions like mine to autoimmune diseases, arthritis, neuropathy, even cancers or diabetes, and injuries—but in pretty much *every* case, there are lifestyle choices we can make to better manage that pain, and to ease it. Our daily choices carry even more weight because those choices have a direct and immediate effect on how we feel physically. We can eat a meal filled with inflammatory foods and pretty much guarantee our pain will be worse in a few hours. Or we can fill our plates and our stomachs with anti-inflammatory foods that can help us feel better and give us more energy. We can win the key battles, and fight our pain by choosing more of the good, less of the bad. This truth has become more real for me than I ever anticipated when I first set out to write this book.

If pain is a reality for you, too, then know that I understand where you are coming from. I get it—man, do I ever. Whether we're talking chronic physical pain, emotional heartache, or mental anguish, I understand. And I want to help you. I want to show you that you can win. Will there be tough days? Yes. But there will be great days too. And I can help you tip that balance in favor of more great days, if you're willing to listen.

If, on the other hand, you picked up this book simply because you want or need to lose some weight, and pain is not a factor, then I can also help you accomplish that. And by taking control of your weight and health right now, you can put yourself on a path toward keeping your body strong in the future. I want you to be able to do life in a body that will carry you wherever you want to go.

The world has changed, and so have our lives, and what we need now is a diet plan that can meet us where we are and help us increase our resilience without depriving us of joy. It's a paradigm shift, really. The old methods of weight loss—the deprivation diets, the hard-core workouts, the high-fat/no-carb or twenty-hour fasting or other unrealistic plans served with a side dish of guilt—none of that is going to help you reach optimal health for your body, at least not in my opinion. The one thing I believe all of those types of diets have in common is that they completely ignore the fact that, even when we're "on a diet," we still have to live our day-to-day lives. We still have to juggle jobs, families, relationships, laundry, and bills; and yes, we still have to carry on when life throws us some kind of crazy curve ball. And that's why I believe a "more of the good, less of the bad" mentality *works*. It's a lifestyle we can adopt and follow for the long haul.

I am so excited to show you how you can embrace this new way of thinking, eating, and living your life to the fullest. This is about so much more than a number on a scale or a waist measurement. This is a mind and body revolution that can put the power of your health back in your hands. So, let's do this. What do you say?

1

THE KICKSTART PHILOSOPHY

The entire premise upon which I'm writing this book is a simple philosophy that I've seen work over and over. It applies to food, exercise, stress, and every other area of our lifestyle. It is a new way of thinking that can help you kickstart your weight and health goals, set you on the right path, and then *keep* you headed in that positive direction. The Kickstart Philosophy is: more of the good, less of the bad.

Notice it's not "only good," or "no bad." Anytime we start thinking in such all-or-nothing terms, we get into trouble. We say, "That's it! I'm finished eating junk food forever. I'm going to live on a steady diet of celery, carrots, and boiled chicken." How long does that last? A day? A week? Two hours? At some point, we find ourselves in the drive-thru line at the local fast food restaurant, ordering a double cheeseburger. Deprivation only serves to make us think more about the things we have sworn off, until we finally give in and indulge. Then we're riddled with guilt that we "failed," and we start to think we'll "never" lose weight and we'll "always" make bad choices. See that all-or-nothing mindset at work? It's really tough to succeed when we are thinking in those terms.

On the other hand, what happens when we give ourselves space to be human? To simply aim for more of what we know is good for us, and less of what we know to be bad for us? We set ourselves up for success.

It removes guilt from the equation, and inspires us to keep going. It helps us to celebrate each victory, rather than browbeat ourselves for a perceived failure. Sounds much more doable, right?

The first question my patients usually ask when we discuss implementing this philosophy in their own life is, "Okay, Doc, it sounds easy enough. But what if your definition of 'good' and 'bad' is different than mine?" It's a great question. These are subjective terms, and it helps to get on the same page regarding their definitions. So, for the sake of clarity, I'm going to give you some specific guidance.

Let's begin with food. This is a diet, after all, and I want you to have a clear understanding of which foods I believe you should be focusing on, and which you shouldn't. I believe that plants are power. I've always known, of course, that vegetables and fruit pack a serious nutritional punch, and that they offer a high amount of fiber, which is great for the gut. Plus, that fiber has a real impact on weight loss. What has really gotten my attention about plants in the past five or so years is what we've learned about just how well they fuel our bodies. We are more able to absorb nutrients from plants, and they have powerful anti-inflammatory properties that help improve overall health.

Now, I'll say this loud and clear several times throughout this book: I am not saying you should consider a fully plant-based diet. I still believe that animal proteins have a place in most people's lives, just not as prominent a place as many folks give them. If I want to have a steak and a glass of wine once a week, I don't see the harm in that. But eating bacon and eggs for breakfast, a turkey sandwich for lunch, and grilled chicken for dinner—well, that is a *lot* of meat. Emerging studies indicate eating that much meat can have a negative impact on our health.[1] Plus, we should consider the environmental factor. Raising meat requires a lot of energy and water, so the less of it we consume, the better it is for our ecosystem.

On the other end of that spectrum, if you're a full-fledged vegan or want to become one, that's great. As long as you're making smart choices about the variety of plant-based foods you're eating, and watching your sugar intake, this can be a sustainable lifestyle for some people.

But I realize it is not for everyone, including me. And that's okay. What I'm saying is that a plant-forward diet plan is beneficial, so the general directive in this book is to reach for more vegetables and fruits.

Which foods should you focus less on? Along with less animal-based protein, I'm going to encourage you to reduce how much processed food you are consuming. By processed, I mean that it's manufactured in some way. If it's sold in a bag, box, or can, it's likely been processed to some degree. And there are plenty of junk foods disguised as health foods on your grocery store's shelves, so we'll beware of those.

Especially in light of the gluten-free, paleo, ketogenic, and other movements, food companies have capitalized on trends and will do anything to sell you on their product as being healthy and even promoting weight loss. I'm not saying they're all terrible for you, only that you should limit your intake of those foods. I frame it like this: eat foods that fuel you, not fool you. That means more whole (unprocessed), plant-forward foods, and less food that has been stripped of its nutrition or manipulated to be something that it isn't. Period.

By the way—have you ever thought about the fact that the acronym for the standard American diet is SAD? And it is pretty sad, really. It's loaded with foods that keep us overweight, tired, addicted, and, well, unhappy. Just check out what most Americans are eating, as reported by the Dietary Guidelines Advisory Committee, which is composed of prestigious researchers in the fields of nutrition, health, and medicine. They calculated that:

> About three-fourths of Americans eat a diet that is low in vegetables, fruits, and beneficial fats.
> Most Americans exceed the recommendations for added sugars, saturated fats, and sodium.[2]

If your own diet reflects this "sad" state of affairs in American eating patterns, don't worry. The changes you will be making can get you on the right track. I know you're running your life at full speed, so let's get you fueled up and ready to race.

I've built the scaffolding of this diet on the foundation formed by *The 17 Day Diet*, a plan that I still believe in wholeheartedly. We've learned a lot about the science of nutrition in the last decade, but the fundamentals that I laid out in that book have stood the test of time. I have heard from thousands of people who changed their own lives using its principles, and it has helped them take command of their health. So I've taken what I've learned and read about in studies, together with feedback from loyal 17 Day dieters and my own patients, and used that information to create the plan you'll read here.

Something else I've become fascinated with in the last couple of years is CBD, or cannabidiol. Perhaps you've heard of it, but you're not sure if it's right for you or even what exactly it does. And I imagine you're wondering what it has to do with weight loss. The bottom line is this: CBD, which you can use in the form of a tincture you ingest or a balm you rub on your skin, has been shown to reduce inflammation and improve sleep, among other benefits that I'll share with you in a chapter on this subject. High-quality sleep is a big key to weight loss. I truly believe that if you changed nothing about your diet or lifestyle for a month except for improving your sleep, you would lose weight. When we're sleeping, our body is doing all kinds of restorative work, and when we aren't getting enough good sleep, those processes are disrupted. This leads to increased hunger, poorer decision-making ability, and a whole host of other side effects that affect our weight. I've had great success with CBD in my own life, and many of my patients and diet testers have too. I can't wait to tell you more about it so that you can start using this incredible tool in your life.

Let's turn our attention to exercise for a moment. As I shared with you in the introduction, I have had times when I forgot my own rule that weight loss and maintenance is 90 percent about the food we eat and 10 percent about the exercise we're doing. In other words, you aren't going to be able to shed pounds if you're exercising like an animal but eating like a college freshman. It just doesn't work that way. But more than that, I want you to move your body for reasons other than weight loss. I want to get you thinking more about keeping your joints lubricated, your spine healthy, and your muscles, ligaments, and tendons flexible, because that's how we prevent a lot of injuries and pain as we age. What happens when we're injured or in pain? We stop moving altogether, and we sometimes turn to food for comfort. Not a great path to be on.

When my patients have gained weight and I ask what's going on, the most common answer I hear is injury. "Doc, I twisted my ankle and now I can't go on my evening walks," or "I hurt my back picking up my kiddo and I can barely get out of bed right now." When I hear that, I say, "Great!" That usually gets their attention. The reason it's great news is that only 10 percent of weight management comes from exercise. So, when you're "broken" in the physical sense, you turn your focus to being as strict as possible on the 90 percent, which is diet. If you follow this plan, the impact of an injury on your weight will be minimal, if any.

Exercise also boosts your immune system. Immunity has become a very hot topic recently, and with good reason. The reason regular exercise is so good for our immune system has to do with circulation. Think about when you drive on the highway. When traffic is flowing, you can get to your destination easily and quickly. Circulation is like highways: the antibodies and all the elements of our blood supply need to get from point A to point B within the body without hitting any traffic on their way to our organ systems. This allows the body's natural healing elements to more easily fight off any pathogens that might be trying to invade. Exercise keeps that circulation flowing without any traffic.

Your brain reaps big benefits from exercise as well. It can boost your mood, improve concentration, and increase mental acuity. There's evidence that it can even help prevent the onset of dementia. So, as you can see, there really are so many reasons to make daily movement a part of your life, and that's why we're going to talk about ways you can move your body more and sit sedentary less. And I want you to have fun while you're doing it, because I know for sure that if it's not fun, you won't do it consistently.

I could fill an enormous gym with the amount of at-home workout equipment my patients are using to hang their clothes on. Why? They don't enjoy using it! But we need to find ways to exercise at home now more than ever, so I'm going to help you unlock the potential for fun and sustainable exercise in the comfort of your house. And while we know a minimum of thirty minutes' worth of physical activity daily is the baseline for good health, I will remind you that it doesn't have to be all at once. Exercise is additive. You could do three sessions of ten minutes, or six sessions of five minutes, or however you want to split it up. Bank those minutes of movement and your body will thank you.

Now, let's talk about stress, which I believe can play a huge role in our weight management. People tend to just throw that word around—"I'm always stressed out," or "Stress is just part of life. It's never going away." I think about it like this. If you said you didn't have any food so you just can't eat at all, that would be a big deal. We'd need to tackle that right away. Or if you couldn't stay hydrated because you didn't have running water, that's a problem we'd need to solve immediately. Right? Well, it's the same with stress. Living in a stressed-out state all the time is detrimental to our health. We do ourselves an injustice if we don't respect it as a serious issue. So let's give stress the respect it deserves.

Chronic stress can hinder our ability to lose weight, because our body is living in a constant heightened state, and it's like we've clicked into survival mode. What does the body do when it's trying to survive? Store fat. Since fat is what the body uses as fuel for many of its functions, we start gaining weight in the form of fat when we're stressed out to the max on a regular basis. Furthermore, stress takes a serious toll on your immune system, leaving you more susceptible to illness.

We'll talk about how to start managing stress on a daily basis so it doesn't stand in the way of weight loss and improved health. I'll share with you my tools for categorizing stress as either "avoidable" or "unavoidable," and then discovering ways to deal with the avoidable stress, and creating coping mechanisms for the unavoidable. And we'll even discuss ways that you can make stress work for you, not against you. I will share with you all my specific "prescriptions" for stress so that you can finally have power over it. I don't want stress to be a roadblock on your path to weight loss and improved health.

There's something else I want to put on your radar that has become a huge topic of conversation in the medical community recently. It's a condition called fatty liver, and it has received quite a lot of attention because it can lead to a deadly condition called cirrhosis of the liver. Now, you might think of cirrhosis as a diagnosis given only to people who abuse alcohol, but the truth is, it can happen to someone who has never had a drop of alcohol in their life. How? Well, a diet full of sugar and unhealthy fats can lead to insulin resistance, which leads to fatty liver disease, which can progress to cirrhosis.

Here's the bad news: cirrhosis is typically irreversible. It often requires a liver transplant, so, yes, it's a very big deal. But the great news is this: fatty liver disease is completely reversible, and it only takes a 10 percent reduction in body weight to do it. So, whether you already have fatty liver or you're at high risk for it, you can absolutely turn it around. Our bodies are amazing, and they respond so beautifully when we give them what they need. How's that for feeling empowered?

I have always believed there are five pillars to good health. They are:

- Nutrition
- Movement
- Stress management
- Hydration
- No smoking

Your goal is always to be moving toward more of the good and less of the bad in all five of those categories; if you do, not only will you lose weight, but your baseline health will improve too.

The bottom line is that you can use this book to accomplish your health goals, no matter what your underlying motivation is. This book is for you if . . .

- You need to lose a significant amount of weight
- You just need to lose those pesky ten pounds that have been hanging around your middle
- You want to boost your immunity and not get sick as often

- You've got a reunion coming up and you want to look amazing
- You've had a rough year (or several!) and you want to get your health back on track
- Your doctor says you're at high risk for fatty liver, diabetes, or cardiovascular disease
- You simply want to feel better and have more energy to do life the way you really want to

As you go through this book and begin to make changes in how you're living, there's one overarching purpose I want you to keep at the top of your mind. Win the key battles. Don't get bogged down with trying to be perfect every day. If you can focus on winning the key battles, you'll begin to see yourself steadily improve. You will lose weight. You will improve your overall health. I've seen patients get off medications they'd taken for years, and have more energy than they did twenty years ago. I've watched people make changes they never dreamed were possible. Here is some inspiration from amazing folks—some of whom have been with me since the release of *The 17 Day Diet*, and others who recently joined our Facebook community—who have been using this plan to lose weight and revitalize their health.

Melissa Erdo says:

"Before finding this plan, I was in pain. I was bloated. I couldn't sleep comfortably. I had heartburn, heel spurs, sinus headaches, and absolutely no energy. Not to mention, emotionally, I was sad and withdrawn. Now, well, I sleep amazing, heel spurs are gone, no more heartburn, no more hot flashes. I'm never sick and I have energy to go all day! Also, I am happy and mentally strong! I see things in a different light. This plan has changed me inside and out."

Lesley Denney says:

"I have more energy and stamina! While at work I would start to drag and feel sluggish after lunchtime, my food usually consisted of fast food; now, with the food change, I have more stamina, feel wide awake, and I can function better at work! Better mindset too. I walk at least five days a week and try to get some cardio in as much as possible. On average I try to do at least sixty minutes of activity a day. This has improved my mobility too! I used to have a lot of aches and pains, take OTC pain pills, now it is rare I need anything!"

I love when people pick up the tools they've been given and use them to create change in their lives. Now it's your turn.

2

KNOW WHERE
YOU'RE STARTING FROM

Your body wants to be healthy. It wants to be in shape and for all of its organ systems to be humming along, working just as they were designed to. For every little bit of encouragement you can give your body in the form of better choices, it will respond accordingly by losing weight, healing itself, and feeling better so you can do life at the pace you want to go. Your body doesn't want to hold you back from the life you truly want to live.

I always tell people who are struggling with weight, if they lose 5 percent of their total body weight, it'll change their life. But if they lose 10 percent of their body weight, it is life-changing. What's the difference? If you weigh three hundred pounds, a 5 percent reduction in weight will change your life in discernible, physical ways. Dropping those fifteen pounds will improve your blood sugars, blood pressure, and fatty liver and it'll give you a better attitude, take away some neck pain, and so on. But a 10 percent reduction in body weight is life-changing in lasting, truly powerful ways. Suddenly you have more confidence. Fatty liver is *reversed*. You realize that you can become an entirely new person, transformed from the inside out. So many things happen at 10 percent.

All of the progress you're going to make on this journey will build upon itself. You can't lose ten pounds without losing one. And you can't form a new daily habit without taking that first step. It all begins by knowing exactly where you're starting from, and I don't just mean the pounds on the scale. I'm talking about the current snapshot of your behavior.

YOUR "GETTING STARTED" QUIZ

Circle your answer to each of these questions below, and then add up your total score. Be honest with yourself, but also know this isn't about sending yourself on a guilt trip. That kind of trip is no fun at all, and usually ends with an extra-large pizza. Remember, where you are today is not where you have to be tomorrow. Your past does not predict your future! For now, let's focus on the present.

1. How often do you currently eat or drink the following categories per week: soda (diet or regular), fast food, fried food?
   - Never—0 points
   - Very rarely, just once in a while—1 point
   - Sometimes—2 points
   - Often—3 points
   - Several times a day—4 points

2. How often do you currently drink alcohol (beer, wine, liquor, alcoholic seltzers)?
   - Never or very rarely—0 points
   - Only on a special occasion—1 point
   - One or two times a week—2 points
   - Three or four times a week—3 points
   - Five-plus times per week on average—4 points

3. How often do you currently eat foods high in sugar (desserts such as ice cream or frozen yogurt, baked goods, candy)?
   - Never or very rarely—0 points
   - Only on a special occasion—1 point
   - One or two times a week—2 points

- Three or four times a week—3 points
- Five-plus times per week on average—4 points

4. How often are you eating plant-forward meals, where animal protein makes up 10 percent or less of the total meal?
   - Every meal—0 points
   - Fairly often—1 point
   - Once in a while—2 points
   - Rarely—3 points
   - Never—4 points

5. What is your current relationship with stress?
   - I'm a zen master; I know exactly how to cope when stress comes—0 points
   - It depends on the day; sometimes I tackle stress head-on, and sometimes I'm a total mess—1 point
   - I worry about the stuff I can't control often, and I feel pretty stressed a lot of the time—2 points
   - A little stress can send me into a tailspin; I have no coping skills that really work for me—3 points
   - I'm a walking stress ball, pretty much in a constant state of fight or flight—4 points

6. On average, how often do you move your body for at least thirty minutes a day, where you work up a sweat?
   - Daily—0 points
   - A few times a week—1 point
   - Once a week—2 points
   - A few times a month—3 points
   - Rarely or never—4 points

7. How much water do you drink each day?
   - 64 ounces (eight 8-ounce glasses) of water or more—0 points
   - Seven 8-ounce glasses of water—1 point

- Six 8-ounce glasses of water—2 points
- Five 8-ounce glasses of water—3 points
- Four or fewer 8-ounce glasses of water—4 points

Scoring

Now it's time to take a look at your answers today and score yourself. Add up your points and write your total score here: _____

0–7 points: You're mastering the "more of the good, less of the bad" philosophy! Keep it up and try to push yourself each day to head toward a 0 score.

8–14 points: You're doing well, and there's always room for improvement. Think of each day as its own challenge to move your score into the 0–7 category.

15–21 points: Your behavior is starting to reflect your desire to make changes in your health, and if you put forth a little more effort, you'll start to experience even more positive results.

22–28 points: Your current lifestyle isn't contributing to your overall health or weight loss goals, but you likely recognize the areas that need your immediate attention, and you have lots of opportunity to celebrate your incremental improvements. You've got this!

No matter what your score is going into this journey, know that this isn't a "cold turkey" type of diet plan. We're not trying to get you from 28 to 0 in the first week. You know as well as I do that that kind of thinking never really works anyway. I want you to embrace this as a way of living that is forgiving, motivational, and adjustable according to your goals. Moving from one group to another on the scoring scale is always rewarding. That's what I always tell my patients: it's not about rushing toward a 0 score, it's just about heading toward better.

You can return to this quiz as often as you'd like while you're working your way through the book and integrating these ideas into your lifestyle. The whole idea is to celebrate your wins and always be on the lookout for simple ways you can make improvements. Your health is dynamic, meaning it changes all the time, so seize each opportunity you have to bring that overall score down!

And there's something else. If you try to think about *all* the main aspects of your health and to make changes across all of them at the same time, it can be overwhelming. Often, it's more doable to focus on one aspect at a time. How do you eat an elephant? One bite at a time. Here's what I mean: let's say stress is a major issue for you. It's a day-in, day-out, constant companion, and you can't remember the last time you got through a day without feeling stressed, anxious, and exhausted. If that's the case, then before you spend one second working on your diet or exercise, you should first focus on managing your stress with the tools I'll reveal in this book. Or if you know in your heart that your food choices are seriously hindering your health and your ability to lose weight, then *that's* your urgent starting point. My point is, you don't need to overhaul your entire life and start from scratch.

Take the Pressure Off

Did you know that for every pound you lose, you take three pounds of pressure off your knees? If you've ever tried to pick up a fifteen-pound bag of rice, you know that's *heavy*! Well, just imagine how much your knees will thank you when you take that much pressure off them when you're walking. That's the benefit you'll experience from dropping just five pounds. The more pressure you can take off the knees, the less wear and tear those vital joints will experience. (See what I did there?) Protecting your joints is a key to being able to stay active as you get older. And as many of my elderly patients will tell you, the biggest factor in aging gracefully is maintaining your mobility! You don't want to live out your golden years having to use a walker or wheelchair. So, do what you can now to help out your knees and hips.

When I talk to folks who used *The 17 Day Diet* to shed pounds, the most common reason they loved it was how quickly they were able to lose weight. It was a "rapid plan," after all! So you might be wondering if you'll experience that same quick weight loss on this diet. The short answer is, yes. If that is your priority, then you absolutely can use this diet to lose weight quickly and safely. It's all about what you put into it. The foods I am specifically recommending will help you burn that stubborn, dangerous visceral fat that collects around your organs. They will also help you reduce bloating. Many of us don't realize that the foods we eat can cause our stomachs to bloat and create uncomfortable gas and digestive problems. If you stick to the nutritional plan I'm outlining, you'll see big improvements in those areas.

HOW YOU'RE FEELING INVENTORY

Right now, let's get a better sense of how you're feeling overall from day to day. Let's assess so we can address! Taking the time to stop and assess how you're feeling is such a valuable exercise. Sometimes it's not until we take a closer look that we realize there are some problem areas to address.

Answer each question in this quiz honestly and thoughtfully. Give yourself a second to think about your average day and how you really feel.

1. Does your stomach feel or appear bloated, especially within an hour or so after eating?
   - Never/very rarely—0 points
   - Sometimes, after a big meal or after foods I know tend to cause gas—1 point
   - Fairly often, at least a couple times a week—2 points
   - A lot of the time—3 points
   - Most of the time/constantly—4 points

2. Do you experience digestive issues such as heartburn, gas, loose stool, constipation, nausea?
   - Never/very rarely—0 points

- Sometimes, especially after I eat or drink specific foods or beverages—1 point
- Fairly often, at least a couple times a week—2 points
- A lot of the time—3 points
- Daily or much of the time—4 points

3. What are your energy levels like?
   - I always have a good amount of energy to complete the tasks I want to, and I have some left over at the end of the day—0 points
   - I run out of steam if I push myself, but for the most part, I have enough energy to sustain me throughout the day—1 point
   - I have sinking spells from time to time, and need to rest during the day—2 points
   - I start to lose energy pretty early in the day, and I struggle to make it through to bedtime—3 points
   - I wake up tired, fight exhaustion all day, pretty much every day—4 points

4. Do you get headaches?
   - Never/very rarely—0 points
   - Sometimes, but usually because I didn't drink enough water—1 point
   - I notice my head hurting, like a dull pain, fairly often—2 points
   - I get debilitating headaches sometimes, and less serious ones often—3 points
   - Headaches have become such a part of my life that I practically put them in my schedule—4 points

5. Do you experience moodiness or mood swings?
   - Never/very rarely—0 points
   - Sometimes, but it's usually hormone-related—1 point
   - I am moody fairly often—2 points
   - My family hides behind the curtains because my mood swings so wildly a lot of the time—3 points

- The least little thing will send me into a tirade . . . and for good reason! The world is driving me crazy!—4 points

6. Do you ever find yourself struggling with lack of motivation?
   - Never/very rarely—0 points
   - Sometimes, but it's usually because something threw me off—1 point
   - Fairly often I find it tough to get motivated to do what I want and need to do in a day—2 points
   - It takes a lot to get me motivated these days; I'd rather just pretend my to-do list is done already—3 points
   - Getting out of bed in the morning is a struggle—in fact, it's noon and I'm still in it right now—4 points

7. Do you ever have trouble focusing, paying attention, or remembering things?
   - Never/very rarely; I'm sharp as a tack—0 points
   - Occasionally I have a case of brain fog, but those are few and far between—1 point
   - I'm noticing this being a problem for me more lately (forgetting where I left my keys, feeling distracted and like I can't focus on the task at hand)—2 points
   - This happens so often that it scares me; my brain just won't hold information the way it used to—3 points
   - What's my name again? And what's this book I'm reading?—4 points

8. How many hours of sleep are you averaging per night?
   - 8+ hours—0 points
   - 7 hours—1 point
   - 6 hours—2 points
   - 5 hours—3 points
   - 4 or fewer hours—4 points

9. How often are you waking up per night?

- Once my head hits the pillow, I'm out until it's time to wake up—0 points
- I might wake up once in a while to go to the bathroom, but it's rare and I can go right back to sleep—1 point
- I wake up occasionally, and when I do, I struggle to go back to sleep—2 points
- I wake up pretty often, and I have to read to fall back to sleep—3 points
- I'm up half the night, restless, unable to string together more than a couple hours of good sleep —4 points

Scoring

0–9 points: Overall, you're likely feeling good, and if there are areas that need improvement, you likely know what those areas are. You can use the tools in this book to feel your absolute best in all areas!

10–18 points: Like all of us, you likely have good days and bad days. Use this assessment as a way to know exactly where to put your energy as you read through this book and begin to implement the tools in your life.

19–27 points: There are probably a couple of areas of your well-being that are feeling off, but once you get focused on them, you will experience serious improvements. You'll soon have specific strategies for each category, and the power to feel better will be in your hands.

28–36 points: You might feel like you're struggling every day, but the great news is that you don't have to struggle anymore. Even improving one area of your overall wellness will have a powerful ripple effect on the rest of your health.

The reason I really want to bring some awareness to your overall well-being, and how you feel throughout the day, is that I think you'll be amazed at how the recommendations I'm making in this book will affect how you feel. Again, this journey is not just about losing weight. It's about having the energy and focus to do your life at the pace you want to go.

There's a great show I started watching on Netflix called *Formula One: Drive to Survive,* and it's a documentary series that takes you behind the scenes into Formula One racing championships. Now, I'm not really all that interested in racing, but this show fascinated me. I had no idea how much goes into just one lap of a race. One lap! It's pure drama. Every single turn is critical. The driver and his or her team have to think about alignment, fuel, overheating, proper maneuvering, tires, the road itself, crashes up ahead, and so on. The same is true for each "lap" of our lives. We live at a furious pace, and we have to be prepared for anything.

Each of us is driving in our own race, and I'm not going to ask you to change that. I think a lot of diet plans overlook the complexity of our individual lives. But you need to be able to get around that lap of life successfully, and do it without "crashing." I'm not going to tell a Formula One driver to slow down around the curve but still win the race. It's not realistic! But what I am going to do is help you optimize your engine, and increase your chances of getting over that finish line without burning yourself out.

HOW'S YOUR LIVER?

If you're like most people, you have no idea how your liver is doing. That's because, unlike other health problems that have clear signs and symptoms, very often, if something's going on with your liver, you'd have no way of knowing. Most people think of alcoholics as being the only at-risk population when it comes to liver disease. But, in fact, there's something called nonalcoholic fatty liver disease, and according to the Mayo Clinic, it affects about one-quarter of people in the US. Yikes—big-time.

This condition occurs when there's too much fat stored in the cells of the liver, and the cause is being overweight. Left unchecked, it can lead to cirrhosis or even death. Not something to be taken lightly. But before you abandon all hope, I'll tell you the silver lining: it's reversible. With only a 3 percent reduction in weight, you slow the process. That means if you weigh two hundred pounds and lose just six pounds, you've already slowed the process of fatty liver disease. With 5 to 7 percent weight loss, you stop it altogether, and with 10 percent weight loss, you begin to reverse the damage. Weight loss is the cure for nonalcoholic fatty liver disease. Isn't that amazing? The power is truly in your hands. So, as you lose weight on this plan, just know that you are doing great things for your liver.

SNAP A PIC

Before we close out this topic on where you're starting from today, I want to try to convince you to take some "before" photos. This will allow you to really become a firsthand witness to the changes your body is undergoing during this diet. It can be for your eyes only, of course. Or if you're the type who loves a good before/after journey, consider sharing it with some friends who can help you stay accountable along the way! It's up to you. But I do encourage you to snap some pictures of yourself, from the front, side, and back. You can have a loved one take them for you, or you can set your phone camera on a timer. You will be so glad you have these so that you can compare and see just how far you've come.

THE 3-DAY "SCRUB"

If there's anything my patients have taught me over the years, it's that they don't like to wait around. They don't want to be stuck in the waiting room, they don't want to wait for lab results, and they *definitely* don't want to wait to lose weight once we start a diet. I get it! One of my favorite lines from a movie was in *The Shawshank Redemption*, when Brooks got out of prison after so many decades, and his first observation was, "The world went and got itself in a big damn hurry." Too true.

When *The 17 Day Diet* came out ten years ago, one of the tag lines I used all the time when I talked about its tenets was, "We can do anything for seventeen days!" Well, now seventeen days can feel like an eternity. So I've made some adjustments to account for that. No, I can't promise to melt away all your excess fat in just twenty-four hours, but what I can do is help you feel and look better in just the first three days. I call it the 3-Day Scrub, because it's all about "scrubbing out" toxins. Think of it like this: if you were converting a garage into a living space, you'd need to thoroughly clean it out *before* you could start moving in a couch, a TV, and a dartboard. You wouldn't want to put your nice couch right on top of a dirty floor stained with motor oil, right?

During the next three days, if you commit to following the specific steps I'm laying out, you are going to be amazed at the changes you will see and feel. On the exterior, you'll see bloating going down, which means a slimming of your waistline, and your weight going down too. On the inside, your body will begin to release toxins, which means your health will already start to improve. The great news is that our organs know exactly how to rid themselves of toxic buildup; all we have to do is eat the foods known to support that detoxifying process.

The 3-Day Scrub can help you break any sugar addiction you might have formed, and rewire those cravings. If you've detoxed from sugar in the past, you might have experienced headaches or other uncomfortable symptoms, but I'm going to give you strategies to help combat those side effects so that you don't feel miserable.

The most powerful way we can help scrub out toxins and begin a health transformation from the inside out is by getting truly hydrated. Even if you're saying, "Hold up, Doc, I already drink enough water to float away," I'll bet you're still not as hydrated as you need to be. This is just another area where "more of the good" comes into play. In *The 17 Day Diet*, I recommended starting your day with a glass of water with fresh lemon. This really gets your digestive system jump-started, but more important, it helps you get into what I call "hydration mode." It doesn't really matter if it's hot, warm, or cold—starting your day with an 8-ounce glass of water, with or without lemon, is always a great idea.

On my private Facebook community called the 17 Day Challenge, I often host something I call Water Wednesday. I ask people to share with me all the different ways they drink water. You'd be shocked at the awesome ideas that come up. Here are a few that they posted:

- "I use a motivational water bottle to track my water intake. It's super easy to follow the time increments and also get the motivational sayings I need throughout the day. I refill at 2 p.m. and by 7, I've had my 64 ounces and anything additional is bonus."

- "I started a practice in college of drinking at least 16 ounces of water first thing after getting up in the morning. I'm also trying to remember to log my water in the Fitbit app."

- "I like to add grated ginger, lemon zest, and lemon to my water."

- "I use little sticky notes with blanks to mark each bottle of water, cup of tea, and my morning lemon drink . . . nothin' fancy!"

- "I have a hiking mug which attaches to my backpack. I live in the high desert, so you can get dehydrated very quickly. Today I drank 80 ounces of H_2O."

- "I fill up my Brita pitcher with 64 ounces of water on the days I'm home all day and keep drinking until it runs dry. I tally on a piece of paper with a pen I keep in my pocket. Simple but it works."

- "I have a water bottle that says 'chug it like it's wine' on it. Ha!"

- "I have eight IKEA plastic cups I put on the counter. As I drink a cup of water, I turn a cup over. Trying to create a new habit!"

Who knew the concept of drinking water could elicit such creativity? I encourage you to join and get some ideas, or share your own.

During the 3-Day Scrub, you'll definitely be increasing your water intake, but you'll also eat foods that boost hydration and do not trigger sensitivities that can cause you to retain water. But this doesn't mean you're going on a liquid diet, not by a long shot. There are plenty of filling, savory foods that you'll be enjoying.

Depending on what your typical diet has looked like up to this point, you will likely be making some radical changes in the next three days. You'll be consuming no sugar or artificial sweeteners, very little or no meat or animal products, no soft drinks or fast food; you'll be replacing all of that with whole, nutrient-dense, healthy options. It might sound somewhat overwhelming, but just stick with me. You can do this.

OKAY . . . WHAT WILL I BE EATING?

I know this is the question at the top of your mind, so let's get right to it. I'm not going to give you a long, boring list of foods you have to choke down at mealtime. There have just been too many times I've walked into the break room at work and seen someone barely able to stand their lunch, and when I've asked what on earth they were eating, they've replied, "Ugh, I don't know. I'm on a diet." That mentality isn't sustainable for long, and I believe a diet that works has to be one that is sustainable, doable, and likable. We've simply got to be able to enjoy what we're eating. And even though the food list isn't super long, I'm confident you'll be able to find enough foods on the list that you like.

THE 3-DAY SCRUB FOODS

These are primarily detoxifying foods to target inflammation and reduce bloating so you'll see a difference right away in how your clothes are fitting. You'll notice there is no dairy and there are no grain-based foods such as bread, crackers, or pasta in this list. I've eliminated those for the first three days because, for some people, those foods can cause bloating and digestive issues. Giving yourself a chance to reset by taking those out of your food rotation helps improve digestion.

You can combine the foods in this list in any way you like, and there are some ideas/inspiration for meals below. Get creative! And even if, at first glance, you don't notice any of your favorite foods here, just approach it with an open mind, and be willing to try some new things. Your body will thank you!

Scrub Food List

- Leafy greens: kale, collards, chard, spinach, bok choy, mustard greens
- Salad greens: romaine lettuce, green leaf and red leaf lettuce, butter lettuce, arugula, endive, baby greens, watercress, dandelion
- Sprouts and microgreens: sunflower sprouts, broccoli sprouts, alfalfa sprouts, daikon sprouts, broccoli microgreens, kale microgreens, mixed microgreens
- Cucumber
- Celery
- Zucchini, zucchini noodles or "zoodles," yellow squash
- Cruciferous vegetables: broccoli (and riced broccoli), cauliflower (and riced cauliflower—there are several commercial frozen versions available), brussels sprouts, cabbage
- Avocado (cut off any brown or black spots, which are caused by oxidation; same goes for any visible mold)
- Tomatoes
- Sweet potatoes, yams, pumpkin, orange squash like butternut and kabocha
- Radishes
- Bell peppers (orange, red, green, yellow)
- Green peas, snap peas
- Green beans
- Asparagus
- Sunflower butter (in moderation: serving amount = 1 tablespoon once a day)
- Pumpkin seeds and pumpkin seed butter (serving amounts = 2 tablespoons unsalted seeds, 1 tablespoon pumpkin seed butter)
- Ground flaxseeds, hemp seeds, chia seeds, sesame seeds
- Quinoa
- Unsweetened flax milk and unsweetened hemp milk
- Canned light coconut milk (½ cup = 1 serving)

- Blueberries, raspberries, strawberries, blackberries, fresh or frozen
- Grapefruit
- Green apples
- Cherries
- Grapes
- Lemon, lime
- Lentils, dal, dried peas
- Chickpeas, hummus (but make sure hummus is oil-free or made with olive oil, no canola or other inflammatory oils—or make your own following the quick recipe on page 38!)
- Tempeh
- Beans: black, pinto, navy, kidney, white, garbanzo
- Pickles, dill relish (no added sugar), sauerkraut (check salt content on all these; it should stay under 100 mg of sodium per serving)
- Fish, especially fish that is low in mercury such as:
  - Sardines, canned in water or olive oil
  - Wild salmon, fresh, smoked, or canned in water (Wild Planet is a good source for high-quality canned sardines and salmon)
  - Rainbow trout
  - Atlantic mackerel
  - Sole
  - Whitefish
- Olive oil (best if drizzled on prepared food rather than used during cooking)
- Avocado oil or avocado oil spray (good smoking point, best choice for cooking oil)
- Apple cider vinegar, raw (such as Bragg)
- Rice vinegar
- Balsamic vinegar
- Coconut oil
- Coconut milk (check ingredients for *no* additives, Native Forest organic unsweetened recommended)

- Coconut water (in moderation)
- Sesame oil
- Soy sauce, tamari, coconut aminos
- Bone broth: chicken, beef, turkey (all low-sodium)
- Vegetable broth (low-sodium)
- Onion
- Scallions/green onion
- Garlic
- Thyme
- Turmeric
- Paprika
- Cilantro
- Oregano
- Ginger
- Chili powder
- Red pepper flakes
- Cumin powder
- Curry powder
- Cinnamon
- Coriander
- Sea salt, Himalayan sea salt, kosher salt
- Black pepper
- Parsley
- Pesto sauce
- Salsa
- Organic green tea, dandelion root and leaf tea, nettle tea, peppermint tea, ginger tea, dandelion "coffee"
- Raw honey (local when possible; 1 teaspoon = 1 serving)
- Organic maple syrup (2 teaspoons = 1 serving)
- 100% whole stevia leaf with no sugar alcohols added (such as erythritol)
- 100% pure monk fruit with no sugar alcohols added (such as erythritol)
- Vanilla extract

That's a pretty robust list, right? And remember . . . three days! That's a lot of food for a three-day stretch. It's true that when it comes to animal-based protein, there's only fish on the menu. But don't worry; I'll add in some optional meats in upcoming cycles. For our Scrub, though, we want to focus on detoxification: you accomplish that with fruits and vegetables. That's the "more of the good" we want!

For this rotation, I'm going to ask you to stick to that list, and only that list. But just in case there's any question about a specific food, I'm also giving you a list of foods that you should avoid while you're on Scrub. The foods on that list are inflammatory foods, dehydrating foods, high-glycemic foods, and refined foods. This is your "less of the bad" list. I'm not saying all of these foods are "bad" in and of themselves; in fact, you'll see some of them in future rotations of this diet. But for just these first three days, we want to give our bodies a break from these so that we can accomplish the first goal of this diet, which is to set the stage for maximum nutrient absorption.

Where's My Chicken?

You might have noticed there's no chicken in the food list for this phase. To be honest with you, I went back and forth on it. I know from *The 17 Day Diet* followers as well as my patients that chicken is a mainstay when it comes to "diet food." It's a lean protein, it's filling, and it can be prepared in a variety of ways. However, when we are trying to really help the body with its natural detoxification processes, chicken can slow us down.

Generally speaking, commercially raised chickens are usually fed corn and soy, and they're usually living in crowded cages, injected with antibiotics to prevent the spread of disease in those close quarters, and so on. This kind of chicken isn't ideal for consuming on a regular basis, because toxins have often accumulated in the meat, and they are then absorbed into our bodies. You can see how that is counterproductive when we're focused on detoxing. So, is there high-quality, free-range, organic chicken out there? Yes, most definitely. You'll pay more for it, but it does exist, and it is better for you.

I always like to make bargains with my patients. And this is an area where I think we can make a bargain. If you simply can't wrap your mind around eating only seafood and plant-based foods for these three days, then you can add in some chicken. I'll even modify some of the recipes to include chicken so you have recipe options. But I'd like you to find free-range, organic chicken that you prepare at home. Nothing that has already been cooked or injected with spices or preservatives—just plain, raw chicken that you cook. Is that a deal? Good!

Foods to Avoid during Scrub

- Beef, pork, lamb, and any other land-animal meat other than chicken
- Shellfish
- Processed meats: deli meats, hot dogs, bacon, sausage
- Processed fake meats: Beyond Burger, Impossible Foods, to-furkey, etc.
- Fast food (anything from a drive-thru is fast food—yes, even the fruit cup)
- Fried foods
- Eggs
- All dairy and all grains
- High-starch veggies: potatoes (other than sweet potatoes), corn, carrots, beets
- Nuts
- Dried fruits
- All artificial sweeteners
- All added sugars (outside of small amounts of raw honey)
- The 3 C's: canola oil, corn oil, and cottonseed oil (because they can cause or contribute to inflammation)
- The 3 S's: soybean oil, sunflower oil, and safflower oil (because they can cause or contribute to inflammation)

STEVIA AND MONK FRUIT EXPLAINED

Artificial zero-calorie sweeteners like aspartame, sucralose (Splenda), and saccharin (Sweet'N Low) are not found in nature; rather, they are synthetically designed in a laboratory. On the other hand, stevia leaf has been consumed for thousands of years. It was traditionally called "sweet treat" and taken as a naturally sweet tea in parts of South America. It has been specifically grown and researched for its natural sweetness for the last hundred years.

Health food stores have been selling stevia for decades, but only in the last decade or so have big food companies gotten in on the act.

However, with stevia being used in a more commercial and processed way, it's really important to note the differences among stevia products. There is whole leaf stevia, the most natural and least processed form; then there are other forms of processed stevia that isolate and concentrate the active compounds known as steviol glycosides. As a general rule, it is better to look for whole stevia leaf and aim to avoid hyperisolated and ultraprocessed forms of stevia like Rebaudioside, which are also manufactured with harsh chemical solvents.

Monk fruit, also known as lo han guo, has been consumed in Asia for centuries. Interestingly, it was first discovered by Buddhist monks. It has been used traditionally as a digestive aid and as a natural sweetener. Monk fruit is a small, round gourd, sort of like a melon. Monk fruit sweeteners are created by removing the seeds and skin, crushing the fruit, and collecting the juice. The fruit extract, or juice, contains zero calories per serving.

Monk fruit has been sold and used mainly as "lo han" for the last several decades, but in recent times, big food companies have started offering more processed versions that are combined with chemicals and alcohols in the lab. There still remains a large handful of smaller companies offering a less-processed, 100% whole monk fruit sweetener.

So here's the key takeaway: stevia and monk fruit are both found in nature—one a leaf, the other a fruit—and have a very long history of use. Now that they have been commercialized, you want to be careful to consume them in their most natural form possible, so look for whole leaf stevia and 100% monk fruit. Sweet!

WHY ARE SOME FOODS INFLAMMATORY?

Many modern diseases that people suffer from are caused by chronic inflammation. To understand what chronic inflammation is, let's first consider acute inflammation. Take an injury, for example. What happens when you're injured? The affected area gets red, warm, and sometimes swollen. That's because your body is responding to the injury and protecting you from infection. After a few days, the signs of inflammation disappear as your injury heals. However, when this kind of inflammation occurs within an organ or organ system, and it doesn't go away, that's considered chronic inflammation. It can be set off by a number of triggers, including stress and food. And it can wreak havoc on your entire body. Some symptoms of chronic inflammation include:

- Headaches
- Irritable bowels (constipation, diarrhea, gas, bloating)
- Tiredness
- Mouth sores
- Generalized pain (joints, chest, abdominal)

That's just a short list; there are many other symptoms that have their roots in chronic inflammation. And left unaddressed, it can lead to serious conditions such as cardiovascular disease, kidney disease, liver disease, arthritis, and more.

There are no two ways about it—sugar triggers inflammation. And if you think artificial sweeteners such as aspartame are a healthy substitute, think again. Your body recognizes aspartame as a foreign intruder, and thus triggers an inflammatory response to it too. I really want to highlight that because sugar and artificial sweetener ingredients are so prolific, and yet so damaging, especially to the work you're doing at the start of these seventeen days.

Here's a list of foods that I consider to be inflammatory:

1. **Sugar and artificial sweeteners:** These can be found in all kinds of places, including candy, milk chocolate, baked goods, soda, diet soda, regular and sugar free ice cream, doughnuts, and sweetened dairy products. Sugar under any other name is still sugar, so here's a list of some of the ways it might show up in ingredient lists on foods:
   - White sugar
   - Fructose

- High-fructose corn syrup
- Corn syrup
- Beet sugar
- Aspartame
- Sweet'N Low
- Splenda (sucralose)

2. **Certain vegetable oils:** Don't be fooled into thinking all plant-based oils are good for you. Some are safe, including coconut oil, avocado oil, and olive oil. But the vegetable oils on this list trigger inflammation in your body:
   - Corn oil
   - Cottonseed oil
   - Canola oil
   - Soybean oil
   - Safflower oil
   - Sunflower oil

3. **Trans fats:** In recent years, there has been a lot of talk about how dangerous trans fats are for you. This refers to industrial trans fats, which are often found in fast food and fried foods. During the manufacturing process, hydrogen is added to the fat. Avoid anything that includes "hydrogenated" or "partially hydrogenated" oil in the ingredient list.

4. **"White" foods:** Foods that are made with bleached flour are also inflammatory. This includes:
   - White bread
   - White pasta
   - Crackers
   - Cakes/pastries

5. **Alcohol:** Especially in excess (more than two servings in a day or seven servings in a week), alcohol of all kinds can be very in-

flammatory. This includes wine, beer, and spirits. I'll go into more depth on this topic later in the book.

YOUR DAILY SCRUB RHYTHM

During these first three days of the plan, you will begin to establish a new daily rhythm. My hope is that you will take this and, over time, customize it to fit your lifestyle. I've intentionally chosen techniques that I have seen work again and again.

1. Begin each day with 12 ounces of warm water with lemon or organic tea. For a little extra flavor and to improve digestion throughout the day, add a little grated fresh or dried ginger to the water or tea.

2. Wait thirty minutes, and then have breakfast. If you don't like eating breakfast or you aren't hungry, it's perfectly fine to wait until lunch. I want you to begin to familiarize yourself with your own body's needs.

3. Try to front-load your day with movement to help your body burn calories and fat efficiently. Go on a walk in the morning, or do some yoga/stretching, or, if you're a gym person, try to get that workout in first thing.

4. Have one snack either midmorning or midafternoon, whichever time you're typically hungrier during the day.

5. Aim to have lunch approximately three to four hours after breakfast.

6. The Rule of 2's: Do not eat fruit after 2 p.m. If you want to lose weight quicker, it's better to eat your fruit earlier in the day. I'll explain more about why later in this chapter.

7. Drink plenty of water in between meals for a total of 64 to 100 ounces of water each day.

8. Have dinner approximately three to four hours after lunch.

9. Try not to eat anything within two hours of bedtime so that your body can use the nighttime for "scrubbing" rather than digesting. Believe it or not, digestion takes a lot of energy, and we would rather your body use that energy in these three days for detoxification.

THE RULE OF 2'S

I'd like to introduce you to a rule of thumb I have been using and recommending for two decades. It's called the Rule of 2's, and it means eating no more than two servings of fruit or starchy carbohydrates (such as sweet potatoes) each day, and *only* eating them before 2 p.m. By consuming your carbs early in the day, you give your body more time to break them down into usable energy. When we eat them past 2 p.m, they become more likely to be stored in the body as fat because we aren't as active. Think about a race car going around a track—does the driver stop to fuel up when there's only a couple laps left? Nope! That would just be dead weight that would slow down the car. It's the same with your body—you don't need that extra fuel in the latter part of your day.

This rule allows you to still enjoy fruit and starchy carbs, but in a way that won't hinder your progress. If you're really intent on losing a lot of weight, and you want to do so as rapidly as possible, you may want to keep this to one serving instead of two. But if you're more focused on feeling better and reducing overall inflammation in your body, then two servings are great. Then, once the clock strikes two, it's all protein and vegetables, which will give you all the energy you need to finish your day strong.

The fruits I'm including in this phase are relatively low in sugar, so if you find yourself craving something sweet later in the day, it's not the end of world if you have a piece of fruit. But as we progress in the plan and add in fruits that are a little higher in sugar, you'll want to start, rather than end, your day with them.

Food Sensitivity vs. Food Intolerance

In the last ten years, as people have gotten more stressed than ever, and more and more people are experiencing symptoms of IBS (irritable bowel syndrome), I've heard a lot of patients say they have food intolerance. Maybe you've even wondered if you are "intolerant" of certain foods. Here's what I want to put on your radar: as with most things, there's a spectrum. There are folks who are completely intolerant of any food with dairy in it. Cheese, ice cream, milk, yogurt—anything with even a hint of lactose (the sugar found in dairy) will cause them gastrointestinal distress. And then there are folks who aren't intolerant, but they are "sensitive" to dairy. Maybe they can't have a big bowl of ice cream, but a cup of yogurt doesn't cause them any issues. They likely have a dairy sensitivity versus an intolerance.

The degree to which you might be sensitive to or intolerant of certain foods can vary widely; the key is to understand your body and know which foods get along with your digestive system, and which ones don't. Bring some awareness to how you feel after you eat "triggering" foods, so that you can adjust accordingly. Also, if you consistently notice uncomfortable symptoms (bloating, cramping, gas, diarrhea, or constipation) every time you eat certain foods, bring it up with your doctor so that you can work together on an effective plan for mitigating your body's response.

Breakfast ideas

- ½ avocado + ½ baked sweet potato + ½ grapefruit
- 1 tablespoon sunflower butter mixed with 2 teaspoons honey, with ½ cup blueberries mixed in

Lunch ideas

- Homemade hummus (chickpeas, turmeric, paprika, olive oil) + cucumber and zucchini "chips" + three-bean salad (mix

three different types of beans for a total of two cups with 2 teaspoons olive oil)
- Smoothie made with coconut milk, frozen blueberries, cinnamon, hemp or chia seeds, 2 teaspoons honey
- Quinoa, green pea, and mixed veggie stir-fry
- Sardines mashed with dill relish, drizzled with olive oil, and seasoned to your liking, atop a bowl of mixed greens (such as arugula, spinach, and butter lettuce)

Snack ideas

- 1 cup bone broth
- ½ cup hummus with cucumbers, celery, or other dipping veggies
- 8 ounces fresh vegetable juice (cucumber, celery, ginger, lemon)
- ½ cup unsalted pumpkin seeds
- Berry cup combining your choice of blueberries, raspberries, strawberries, and blackberries, topped with a dash of cinnamon

Dinner ideas

- Veggie chili made with beans, zucchini, bell peppers, chili powder, diced sweet potato
- Avocado/cilantro salad atop arugula, sprinkled with lemon juice and topped with 6 ounces of broiled chicken
- Steamed salmon with zucchini "boats" baked with hummus, paprika, and garlic, topped with sunflower seeds
- Lentil soup made with bone broth and diced veggies + baked kale chips

Feel free to mix and match the foods in the Scrub food list as much as you'd like. Find those flavor combinations that work for your palate. Think of the vegetables on the list as foods that you can eat with abandon. The fiber from those veggies makes them so filling, and great for the gut, so I'm not concerned about you overdoing it.

You might be wondering about overall portion sizes, especially if you're someone who tends to "go big." Here's what I tell my patients: the protein in your meal should be the size of your whole hand, from the base of your palm to your fingertips. With the nonstarchy vegetables, as I mentioned, you can go crazy, so don't worry about a specific portion size on those. And when you do introduce a starchy vegetable, or another carbohydrate, think of just the palm of your hand as a guide for that portion size. Now, keep in mind: that doesn't mean it can be the size of your palm, but stacked six inches high like a short stack of pancakes. Fold your fingers over to where they're just about touching your palm, and there's a little pocket that forms. That's the portion size we're going for.

I like to strategize each meal, and while it may sound funny, it really works. For the first few bites of the meal, I only eat the protein and vegetables. I eat pretty slowly, allowing the food to hit my stomach so those satiety signals can set in. Very often, the only food left on my plate at the end of the meal is the starch, because I got full before I could eat it all. It's a great little trick for filling up on the healthiest foods on your plate!

GET SPICY

Healthy food gets a bad rap as being bland or tasteless. But it doesn't have to be that way! I want you to fling open the doors of your spice cabinet and start experimenting with spices and herbs. They can really dress up vegetables. Here are a few ideas:

- **Rosemary:** This herb is delicious with roasted potatoes, onions, or cauliflower, with beans or Italian dishes. It smells and tastes so good, fresh or dried, and it's also a powerful antioxidant.

- **Garlic:** A relative of onions and shallots, garlic packs a tasty wallop. Dice it up for a salad dressing, or sauté it with mixed veggies.

- **Dill:** Fresh dill added to steamed broccoli or green beans is a fantastic combination. It's also great with fish, carrots, and cucumbers.

- **Cinnamon:** This spice has great health benefits, including giving a boost to our metabolism. It tastes great with all types of fruit, and even infused in your water or sprinkled in your coffee.

- **Lemon:** You know I love fresh lemon squeezed in water, but it's also delicious squeezed into salad dressing, or on top of vegetables. Furthermore, lemon rind is a great antioxidant, so consider grating it over a salad.

- **Mustard:** Dijon mustard adds a lot of flavor to chicken, fish, or even a vegetable dish. Just make sure that you're reaching for one that doesn't have a lot of extra sugar, as honey mustard does.

- **Mint:** Mix this delightful herb into a smoothie, or into a bowl of fresh berries.

- **Basil:** Tomato-based dishes always taste great with basil added, as do chicken dishes. Plus, it's easy to grow in pots, so you can always have some on hand.

TO THE SALT FIENDS

If you love putting salt on your food, or if your cravings tend toward the salty/crunchy category (potato chips, french fries, salty popcorn, and the like), then let's have a little chat. First, you should be aware that a high quantity of sodium is dehydrating, so it can thwart all the efforts you're making toward better hydrating yourself and even cause water retention. And especially during these first three days of the plan, when you are doing your best to detoxify your body, hydration is critical. Plus, in the long term, a diet that's super high in sodium can lead to high blood pressure and other serious health concerns.

You weren't born loving salt. It's a taste you acquired over time. And as such, you can learn to love other flavors even more. Throughout this eating plan, you will find a lot of fresh and dried herbs and spices, all of which are bursting with flavor. By using less salt, you will begin to truly taste and appreciate the flavors in your food. Become more mindful about tasting food as it was meant to be enjoyed, and connecting the taste of the food with the benefits it has for your body.

Now, with all of that said, I don't want you to think that the only way to succeed is to go salt-free. On the contrary, salt in moderation can be very beneficial, especially if you opt for sea salt. It is packed with trace minerals, which can be tough to come by these days because much of our produce is grown in soil that isn't as nutrient-rich as it once was. Sea salt can also help improve digestion and absorption of vitamins from food. So, don't swear off the salt altogether, but do choose it wisely and use it sparingly.

M&M (NO, NOT THE CANDY!)

M&M stands for mindfulness and motivation, a concept I talk about with my patients daily. Oftentimes, we lose our focus, or forget our reason for working so hard to improve our health. But if we don't keep what's driving us in mind, we easily lose sight of our goal. What's your motivation? Are you retiring in the next couple years and you want to feel good enough to travel with your companion? Do you have kids or grandkids you want to be able to play with? Are you trying to get off some or all of your medications? Is your high school reunion coming up, and you want to be able to walk in feeling strong and confident? For me, I want to do everything I can to reduce the amount of pain I experience so I can show up as the best possible version of myself for my patients. That's what keeps me going. Whatever it is that's motivating you to lose weight and reclaim your health, I want you to keep that front and center as you continue. Write it down, keep it in your phone, or post it on your fridge, in your car, or wherever you might need a gentle reminder of that motivation.

Vicki's Story

I developed this entire diet by listening closely to a loyal (and huge!) group of people who found success on the 17 Day Diet. They have been offering feedback along their own journeys, and I've leaned into that feedback during the creation of this program. I've shared the recipes, foods lists, and overall philosophy of this new plan with them, and they've truly helped me shape it every step of the way. So, when I asked the 17 Day Diet challengers to share with me some of the success they've had with this specific program, Vicki's response was just awesome! Here's what she said in her own words:

"I am a true believer that this program saved my life. I turned sixty in August of 2020. And while this year in particular has been a difficult year for our world, I will always remember 2019 and 2020 as the years I took back my life. I went through terrible back pain in 2019. Dr. Mike's words and this program taught me to focus on what I could do. I did just that and never looked back. I went from barely being able to do stretches given to me from a physical therapist to walking sometimes up to seven or eight miles in one day without it fazing me. I set out with one focus: to get as healthy as I possibly could. And not to grow old relying on a fistful of pills to get me through a day. After all, I have grandkids to enjoy! In the process, pounds and inches (fifty-four inches in total) started falling off. As my physical ability changed, my confidence improved. I want to reach as many people as I can with my story. They need to know there is an answer that isn't ridiculously expensive or difficult to follow. So I share information wherever or whenever a conversation

Vicki's story and all of the others like hers are so inspiring. This is why I love doing this. Way to go, Vicki!

Bringing some mindfulness to your decisions is the other aspect. If you take five seconds before grabbing that muffin from the coffee shop to check in with yourself, to remind yourself of what's motivating you, then you're probably not going to order the muffin. Give yourself that chance to make the decision that keeps you on track. *That's* being mindful. It doesn't take a lot of effort. Will you sometimes still go with the muffin and not look back? Sure. That's okay too. But at least you were mindful about it, and you made the conscious decision instead of just going with a knee-jerk reaction and then regretting it later.

The other day, I got home from work and I was beat. Often when I'm frustrated or I've had a long day, I just want to go to a restaurant, relax, and get my mind off it. But I took a minute, and I said to myself, *I can do that, or I can just put on my swimsuit, go down to the pool, and swim 1,500 yards.* That's what I did. Afterward, I was so happy. I had gotten in thirty minutes of swimming, which made me more energetic, and then I went to the fridge and made a beautiful, delicious salad. My mindset had changed. The choice derailed my negative pathway. Plus, I saved myself $100 by not going out to the restaurant! The satisfaction I felt was so much more than if I'd gone out. So, you see, I don't just make this stuff up; I actually do it!

I use this same tool a lot with patients who are trying to quit smoking. When they feel like reaching for a cigarette, I tell them to reach for a glass of water and a five-minute walk instead. When we're feeling tempted, I think we need to get up and move. So, anytime you're struggling to fight off a craving, try drinking a glass of water and going for a quick walk, even if it's from one side of your house to the other. It's similar to approaching a speed bump—instead of just barreling over it and getting all shaken up and out of alignment, slow down and let each tire get over the bump. We do less damage that way!

You're not going to win every battle, but here's what I want you to remember. Just like in sports, you don't need to be undefeated in order to win the championship. You just need to win some key games. By being mindful, you are at least giving yourself a chance to get a win. The more you win, the better you get.

Will there be crazy days when everything seems to be going wrong, you're stressed to the max, and you just give in left and right to every temptation? Yep. But there's always a second half. Think about a professional sports team that prepares for a game—the players watch film, study players, practice until all hours—and then on game day, they're outmatched. By halftime, they're getting crushed, and they're like, *What happened*?! It's exhausting and demoralizing, and it bums you out. There's always a second half. Pick up the pieces, look at what you did right, and look at what you can improve upon. You still have that second half of your day to make a few right decisions and potentially win. It's about that recognition, taking a moment, and you will start to win more than you lose. *Awesome*!

Beating Those Sugar Withdrawals

As I touched on earlier, if you're used to consuming quite a bit of sugar on a daily basis, you might feel some withdrawal effects in these three days. Sugar can be a very real addiction, so those side effects are very real too. But remember, it's only temporary. And here are some tips for feeling better if you experience lethargy, headaches, or tummy upset as a result of sugar withdrawals:

1. **Pack in the Protein:** Having a high-protein snack can give you energy and help ease symptoms. A few nuts, some seeds, or a tablespoon of sunflower butter can do the trick.

2. **Fix It with Fiber:** Vegetables that are high in fiber are always a good idea for a snack because fiber can help regulate blood sugar. Try half an avocado, a baked sweet potato, some sliced radishes, or a couple servings of roasted asparagus.

3. **Ginger to the Rescue:** Add some fresh or powdered ginger to a cup of herbal tea and reap the benefits of this long-celebrated root. Ginger can soothe the stomach and help with headaches.

4. **Try Some Acupressure:** If you have a withdrawal headache, gently squeeze the area of your hand between your thumb and index finger, and then pulse it for two minutes. You might be surprised at how much better (and quicker) this can work than an over-the-counter headache medication. Definitely try this before popping a pill.

5. **Water, Water, Water:** There's no greater fix for sugar detox symptoms than water. The dilutional effect is so powerful. Imagine it washing those sugar toxins away with every sip.

BUT FIRST, COFFEE . . . RIGHT?

Ah, coffee. One of the main questions I get from people is whether they can have their morning cup of joe. Look, the short answer is yes. But there are a couple catches. First, I said coffee, not a caffé mocha with three shots of espresso, whipped cream, and chocolate drizzle on top. Clearly, that's not going to work here. And even a "dash" of cream or a "tiny bit" of sugar is not part of the equation for right now. If you really need coffee, I recommend drinking it black and limiting it to one cup. (I know, I know, so boring.)

Coffee is dehydrating; there's no two ways about it. I always have to chuckle when I ask my patients if they are drinking enough water and they answer, "Yes!" (Pause.) "Coffee counts, right?" Actually, no, coffee doesn't count. In fact, I think of coffee as "negative water," meaning for each cup you drink, you have to drink one cup of water to replace it. That's completely fine, as long as you end up at a positive 64 ounces of water at the end of the day.

Instead of coffee, I'd suggest starting your day with a cup of organic tea. Green tea has only about one-third the amount of caffeine that coffee does, but it will give you a slow, steady state of energy rather than the peaks and valleys coffee can create. But if you're in a committed relationship with your coffee, just counter it with plain water.

Here's another heads-up: if you're detoxing hard off a high-sugar diet, then I can guarantee caffeine is only going to make matters worse. The more you can flush out your system with pure water, the fewer negative symptoms you're going to experience, such as headaches and sluggishness. I know it seems simple, but water really is your best friend for these three days.

IS FASTING THE FAST TRACK TO WEIGHT LOSS?

There's been a lot of buzz around intermittent fasting in recent years, and for good reason. Research indicates that fasting, when done properly, can have significant health benefits, including better glucose control in diabetic patients.[3] But will it help you melt fat? Well, there is some evidence that it could moderately improve weight loss efforts, but it's not a silver bullet by any stretch.

So you might be wondering if I'm recommending any fasting for this diet. Overall, I'm a fan of the concept of intermittent fasting. I think it's generally a good idea to eat all of your meals in an eight-hour window and then fast for sixteen hours. It gives your body a chance to spend energy on vital processes aside from digestion. But I'm not requiring it because I don't think it's super realistic for most people.

Should you decide to try out intermittent fasting and see how it agrees with you, keep in mind your activity level and schedule. If you tend to work out early in the morning and then start your day, skipping breakfast might be a challenge. Whatever residual energy you have from the previous day, you're going to spend it on that workout. You might feel calorically deprived until lunch. Also, some people have hypoglycemic tendencies; if that's you, then pay extra attention to how you're feeling during a fast. If you're starting to have symptoms such as dizziness or light-headedness, definitely break the fast with a healthy snack.

I've never been a breakfast person, so I often fast without even thinking about it. I exercise at lunch, so in the morning, I get up, have my coffee or green tea, drink about 50 ounces of water, and start my day. I'm good to go through my workout, and then I enjoy lunch. So, who are you? Are you a morning workout person? Noon? Or night? Schedule your fasting and eating windows around your activity so that you have enough energy in the form of food to fuel you.

PLAYING THE "HUNGRY" GAMES

Anytime you start eating in a different way, your body goes through an adjustment period. Part of that adjustment has to do with acquainting yourself with unfamiliar hunger signals. You might be used to feeling hungry at certain times of the day, or your hunger might be triggered by emotional responses such as stress, boredom, or fatigue. During the first week or two of this diet, those feelings of hunger might be showing up with more or less intensity, and at different times of the day than usual. Give yourself a chance to notice them, to get used to them, and to always address them first by drinking water. That's right: very often, when we think we're hungry, we're actually thirsty. So, first, drink 8 ounces of water, wait ten minutes, and then reevaluate to see if you truly need a snack or your next meal.

Generally, it's smart to wait about four hours between meals. That gives your body time to fully digest and put those nutrients to good use before you're filling up again. If you just can't make it to the next meal, I'm including snack ideas in each phase of the diet. I don't love to give food options in "unlimited quantities" for between meals, because if we know there are some foods that we could eat all day long, then we tend to do just that—eat all day long. And that's not a great idea, even if you're eating cucumber slices and steamed spinach from sunup to sundown. The idea is to get your body into a healthy rhythm between eating and resting so that you can begin to self-regulate how much food you're consuming each day. But if you do feel like you're about to keel over at some point, always feel free to grab a life preserver such as a hard-boiled egg, a couple of pickle spears, a handful of berries, or a few nuts to tide you over.

For some people, tracking their hunger is helpful. You might want to write down how hungry you feel when those first pangs set in, and then you can decide if you might need to add a bit to your breakfast or lunch so you can make it to the next meal without feeling like you could swallow an elephant whole. If you do track your hunger, use a scale of 1 to 5, with 1 being barely hungry at all and 5 being ravenous. Then, as you adjust your meals accordingly, see how those numbers change the next day and the day after. Before you know it, you'll be able to go four hours between meals just fine.

CHANGING BOWEL HABITS

Anytime we make changes to our diet, we are likely to experience changes in our bowel habits. Everyone is different; some people may experience constipation, others may have diarrhea. Maybe you won't experience noticeable changes at all. But I bring this up so that you can be aware and prepared.

We're adding in a lot of fiber and a lot of hydration, and those two factors right there can have a significant impact on your overall digestion. What I tell my patients is to give themselves a seventy-two-hour time frame to adjust. Detoxification happens primarily in the colon. It's where the absorption of water takes place, in the sigmoid colon. If you're drinking plenty of water, your colon will be happy because it won't have to work overtime to squeeze water out of your food. If you do start to feel constipated, try drinking more water—that can make a big difference.

You can think of any alteration in your bowel habits as evidence of change, and that's inspiring. It's your body's way of thanking you for making healthier choices.

READY TO SOAK UP

We are all starting from a different place anytime we begin a new diet program. As a result, some people may have a very dramatic transformation in the first three days, and others might not experience as big a shift. If you're starting from a place of just being a little bit off the path, then your changes might not seem as dramatic to you. But here's what I want you to know: the foundation you are laying in these first three days is solid. It is setting the stage for a new level of wellness in your life. Don't allow yourself to get discouraged if you don't lose five pounds and a pants size in three days. Understand that the transformation is occurring on a cellular level, and the physical results will come. And it won't take long.

If you're experiencing the effects of carbohydrate withdrawal, hang in there. The Scrub can really pack a wallop for a hard-core carboholic. You might feel gastrointestinal disturbances, headaches, fatigue, and intense cravings. Use the tools I've given you in this chapter and know that those side effects are proof that your body is detoxifying. They are a good sign! This is just seventy-two hours. It's *so* doable.

Once you're all "scrubbed," and you've enhanced your body's natural detoxification process, you are primed and ready to "soak up" some of the best nutrients Mother Nature has to offer. You've laid important groundwork here, and you've switched your body and mind into a new mode. Keep up the great work, and let's continue on this exciting journey together.

4

THE 4-DAY "SOAK UP"

Congratulations on completing the first three days! You should know—you've just made it through the toughest part. And you've laid the important groundwork for self-confidence because you've shown yourself what you can do when you put your mind to it. You are actively getting your health to a better place. With any goal we're seeking to achieve in life, our belief in our ability to acquire that goal is the most important indicator of success. You've shown yourself what you're capable of, so let's tackle this next phase with gusto!

Over these next four days, you're going to be loading up your body with all kinds of phytonutrients, which are specific chemicals found only in plants. They interact with the vitamins and minerals to protect the body, fight free-radical damage, and aid in the prevention of disease. Antioxidants, polyphenols, and carotenoids are some common examples of phytonutrients. A simple way of thinking about phytonutrients is color: the more colorful the food, the more phytonutrients! And because of the work you've already done, your body will accept, absorb, and utilize all of these supercharged antioxidants, vitamins, and minerals better than ever. You will likely experience improved mental acuity, clarity, and memory as well as a burst of energy, plus a flatter tummy and reduced digestive issues.

We'll also put a greater emphasis on foods like sauerkraut (which was in the first phase) and kimchi, because they offer naturally occurring probiotics.

If you're worried about feeling hungry, don't be. Sensible snacking is allowed, and I will provide you with a list of snacks that will satisfy you. I don't believe you have to feel hungry all the time in order to lose weight; in fact, allowing yourself to get too hungry can switch on cravings in your brain, and you set yourself up for making poor choices. So this phase is designed to help you feel full and satisfied.

WHAT ABOUT EXERCISE?

You might be wondering where exercise fits in. (Or maybe you were afraid to ask.) Here's the deal. The Scrub phase is like when the service light goes on in your car and you're a little nervous about driving it around town until you can take it into the shop. You know you need to have the filters changed, the tires rotated, belts replaced, fluids topped off, and everything under the hood checked out. That's essentially what you've just done in the first three days of this plan. You took your body in for service. Just like when you pick up your car from the shop and you can't wait to take it out for a spin, now that your body is functioning properly, you can begin to exercise.

You might have felt a bit sluggish for the first three days. Maybe you had a couple headaches and your body just didn't feel exactly right. That was because your body was spending so much energy on detoxification. It was releasing some of those stored-up toxins, which takes some adjustment. But in these next four days, your energy levels should return and your uncomfortable symptoms should dissipate. It's the perfect time to begin to include some mild exercise.

I recommend starting slowly and working your way up. If you have exercise bands at home, use those for some gentle stretching and resistance moves. Focus on stretching your hamstrings and lower and upper back. I want you to take deep, cleansing breaths with each move, and become aware of your body in a new way. The goal isn't to rush to a sweat, or to burn 1,000 calories. We are forming a new habit, one in which you exercise with mindfulness, so that it can be more effective and have longer-lasting results. And at first, we are just testing things out to see how you feel. It's that first drive around the block.

Let that body awareness be with you throughout the day, not just when you are intentionally exercising. Movement is not something we should do for just thirty minutes or an hour each day—it is a state we should be in for the majority of our waking hours. Think about how you are sitting at your desk or on the couch. What is your posture like? Are you engaging your core muscles when you move? When you walk, are your shoulders back so that your chest opens up and you're able to breathe more deeply into your lungs? Are you standing up often enough and stretching your back so that you can get the blood flowing? Even doing ankle circles while you watch television can be incredibly helpful in keeping your ligaments healthy and your joints lubricated.

Slowly, between now and the end of the first seventeen days of this plan, begin to increase the length and rigor of your exercise routine. That might mean going from five minutes of stretching and one lap around your block to fifteen minutes of stretching and a two-mile walk. Or that could mean going from thirty minutes in the gym doing resistance training to an hour of cardio and resistance. In a later chapter, I'll give you tons of ideas for incorporating movement into your lifestyle in fun ways. For now, just think about moving more and sitting less!

Throughout this phase, as you continue to properly hydrate and fuel your body, one exciting aspect is that you're going to be less prone to injury. Hydration has a surprisingly big impact on injury. When you look at the musculoskeletal system and its ability to function and perform, hydration is critical—it helps you experience fewer of those "service lights" along the way. So, if you've struggled with exercise-related injuries in the past, my hope is that you'll notice fewer issues going forward.

Soak Up Food List

Note: You can eat all of the foods from the 3-Day Scrub Food List, which are:

- Leafy greens: kale, collards, chard, spinach, bok choy
- Salad greens: romaine lettuce, green leaf and red leaf lettuce, butter lettuce, arugula, endive, baby greens, watercress, dandelion
- Sprouts and microgreens: sunflower sprouts, broccoli sprouts, alfalfa sprouts, daikon sprouts, broccoli microgreens, kale microgreens, mixed microgreens
- Cucumber
- Celery
- Zucchini, zucchini noodles or "zoodles," yellow squash
- Cruciferous vegetables: broccoli (and riced broccoli), cauliflower (and riced cauliflower), brussels sprouts, cabbage
- Avocado (cut off any brown or black spots)
- Tomatoes
- Sweet potatoes, yams, pumpkin, orange squash like butternut and kabocha
- Radishes
- Bell peppers (orange, red, green, yellow)
- Green peas, snap peas
- Green beans
- Asparagus
- Sunflower butter (in moderation; serving amount = 1 tablespoon once a day)
- Pumpkin seeds and pumpkin seed butter (serving amounts = 2 tablespoons unsalted seeds, 1 tablespoon pumpkin seed butter)
- Ground flaxseeds, hemp seeds, chia seeds, sesame seeds
- Quinoa
- Unsweetened flax milk and unsweetened hemp milk

- Canned light coconut milk (½ cup = 1 serving)
- Blueberries, raspberries, strawberries, blackberries, fresh or frozen
- Grapefruit
- Green apples
- Bananas
- Lemon, lime
- Lentils, dal, dried peas
- Chickpeas, hummus (make sure hummus is oil-free or made with olive oil, no canola or other inflammatory oils—see your quick homemade recipe!)
- Tempeh
- Beans: black, pinto, navy, kidney, white, garbanzo
- Pickles, dill relish (no added sugar)
- Fish, especially fish that is low in mercury such as:
  - Sardines, canned in water or olive oil
  - Wild salmon, fresh, smoked, or canned in water (Wild Planet is a good source for canned sardines and salmon)
  - Rainbow trout
  - Atlantic mackerel
  - Sole
  - Whitefish
- Olive oil (best if drizzled on prepared food rather than used during cooking)
- Avocado oil or avocado oil spray (good smoking point, best choice for cooking oil)
- Apple cider vinegar, raw (such as Bragg)
- Rice vinegar
- Balsamic vinegar
- Coconut oil
- Coconut milk (check ingredients for *no* additives; Native Forest organic unsweetened recommended)

- Coconut water (in moderation)
- Sesame oil
- Soy sauce, tamari, coconut aminos
- Bone broth: chicken, beef, turkey (all low-sodium)
- Vegetable broth (low-sodium)
- Onion
- Scallions/green onion
- Garlic
- Thyme
- Turmeric
- Paprika
- Cilantro
- Oregano
- Ginger
- Chili powder
- Red pepper flakes
- Cumin powder
- Curry powder
- Cinnamon
- Coriander
- Sea salt, Himalayan sea salt, kosher salt
- Black pepper
- Parsley (which really helps with detoxification)
- Pesto sauce
- Salsa
- Organic green tea, dandelion root and leaf tea, nettle tea, peppermint tea, ginger tea, dandelion "coffee"
- Raw honey (local when possible; 1 teaspoon = 1 serving)
- Organic maple syrup (2 teaspoons = 1 serving)
- 100% whole stevia leaf with no sugar alcohols added (such as erythritol)
- 100% pure monk fruit with no sugar alcohols added (such as erythritol)
- Vanilla extract

New foods:

- Dark chocolate (70% cacao or higher; 1 serving = 1 ounce)
- Cacao (powder or nibs)
- Eggs (free-range, organic)
- Mushrooms
- Carrots
- Beets
- Artichoke
- Seaweed
- Basil (fresh)
- Rosemary (fresh)
- Kimchi
- Pickled ginger
- Pickles (look for pickles with no added sugar)

Note: You may eat chicken as needed, just like in the Scrub phase.

Soak Up Snacks

In these four days, you might notice more hunger pangs here and there, especially as you begin to increase your activity levels. If you're feeling hungry between meals, I'm listing some snacks you can grab, within moderation. I'm including serving sizes here so there's no guesswork on your part.

- Berries (strawberries, raspberries, blackberries, blueberries): ½ cup
- Boiled eggs: 2
- Pickles: 2
- Celery: 1 cup, diced
- Jicama: 1 cup, diced (add a dash of lemon or lime juice)
- Carrots: 1 cup

YOUR DAILY SOAK UP RHYTHM

During the first three days, you got into a new daily rhythm. During the Soak Up phase, you'll continue to build on that routine.

1. Begin each day with 12 ounces of warm water with lemon or organic tea. Add ginger if desired.

2. Wait thirty minutes, and then have breakfast. Or if you prefer, you can wait to eat your first meal of the day until lunch. Hopefully you're starting to get in tune with your body's natural cycle of hunger and satiety.

3. Find ways to work in some movement, or do your daily exercise routine early in the day if possible.

4. Enjoy one snack either midmorning or midafternoon, whenever you're typically hungrier.

5. Aim to have lunch approximately three to four hours after breakfast. Allow your body to get hungry, but not ravenous, before eating.

6. Remember the Rule of 2's: No fruit or starches after 2 p.m.

7. Drink plenty of water all day long.

8. Enjoy dinner approximately three to four hours after lunch.

9. Avoid eating within two hours of bedtime.

TRACK YOUR FOOD CHOICE PROGRESS

Journaling is a powerful activity. I've journaled a lot over the past several years, and it has been instrumental in my physical and emotional recovery. Journaling can help you work out how you're feeling physically as well as emotionally, in correlation to what's happening in your life—the good, the bad, and the ugly. This is all valuable data that can help you connect dots and see behavioral patterns.

If you don't already keep a journal, I encourage you to begin. You don't have to write a novel with every entry; it can just be a few lines at the end of each day. Or even every two or three days. It can be a very revealing, and even cathartic, exercise.

There's another way that journaling can be beneficial to you, and that's in your relationship to food, especially foods that you know you shouldn't be consuming on a regular basis. We're all familiar with the term *guilty pleasures*. We know we shouldn't indulge, but for whatever reason, sometimes we do anyway. I'm not here to make you feel more guilty, because that's counterproductive; but what I do think we should work toward is being honest with ourselves about how often we're giving in to these foods, so that we can begin to rein that in. Again, the goal isn't perfection here. I'm not saying we should try to never again give in to the call of a bear claw. But we should aim to give in a little less often.

So, just how many times a week do you eat something you know isn't doing your body any favors? Maybe it's soda, or perhaps potato chips. I won't go down the list of endless possibilities, because you already know exactly what your Achilles' heel is. Now it's time to get honest with yourself about how much of it you're consuming.

I know most of us don't *mean* to deceive ourselves or our doctors when they ask about our habits. But when we are racing around that lap of life, we've got a lot going on, and it's harder for us to recognize our own behaviors. We have so much on our minds that we don't often stop to think about how much we're actually indulging in guilty pleasures. So, we estimate. But if you are like me, that estimate is usually lower than the actual number. We can't deal with what we don't know, so let's use journaling to gain some knowledge about our habits.

In the first column of the chart below, write down the foods you tend to eat but know you shouldn't. Then think about how often you've been indulging in them lately. My hope is that you've been able to swear them off for the last three days, but think back to the previous month leading up to you starting this plan. Were you eating two servings, twice a day? One serving, once a week? Write it down in the second column.

Then, one month from now, come back to this chart and fill in the third column. Your goal is for the numbers in that third column to be lower than in the second column. I think you'll be surprised how easy it becomes over time, because you won't even be thinking about those foods anymore. Let's see!

Guilty Pleasure Food	How Much and How Often I Currently Indulge	How Much and How Often I Indulge after 30 Days

Now, let's look at the other side of that coin. Think about ten healthy foods that you know you should be eating more of, but you currently aren't eating that often. This might be a really easy exercise for you, or it might be tough. If you're not sure where to start, just take a look back at the food lists for these first two phases of the diet. Maybe there's something on one of those lists you've never even tried before. Or perhaps you've had a couple of them before, and didn't think you liked them. Are you willing to give them a second chance? Start with a clean slate? Or maybe there was a healthy food you used to love, but you sort of forgot about. Put them all on the list.

As you move through this plan, I want you to start incorporating more of the foods that we know nourish your body, such as vegetables, fruits, and fish; that's why it's smart to get very intentional about it by listing the foods you want to focus on. Then write down how often you're currently eating each of those foods. And finally, thirty days from now, return to this chart and fill in how often you're eating them at that point. By putting it at the forefront of your mind and challenging yourself to increase your intake of these foods, you'll greatly increase the odds of actually doing so. Plus, as you try them more, you'll begin to rewire your taste buds in such a way that you will find yourself looking forward to eating these foods the way you used to look forward to your guilty pleasures.

Healthy Food	How Much and How Often I Currently Eat It	How Much and How Often I Eat It after 30 Days

MY NEW PATIENT HERO

My patients very often become my heroes. I get so inspired by their stories of transformation and motivation. So when I recently met Frank (not his real name, but his story is true), I just had to share it with you because I knew it would inspire you too.

I looked down at my schedule the other day and noticed I had a new patient. After twenty-five years of practicing as a general physician, that doesn't happen very often anymore. My panel, as it's called, is pretty much closed, and I have my regular patients that I see. But Frank was changing MDs, and I had some space in my schedule. I read over his details, and saw that he's ninety-four years old. It was surprising that someone that age was opting to change doctors. I wondered what was up with that. I was a little concerned that perhaps this was going to be a complicated case.

Later that afternoon, it was time for Frank's appointment. When I swung open the door and saw him sitting there, I thought maybe I'd entered the wrong room. This guy couldn't be ninety-four! He was seventy-five if he was a day. Well-groomed, fit, and sitting up straight and alert, Frank looked back at me, smiled, and cheerfully said, "How do you do, Doctor?"

We chatted for a while, and it turned out Frank has something we refer to as "white-coat syndrome," and that was part of why he'd wanted to changed doctors. Every time he would go in for an appointment, his blood pressure typically shot up, and it was purely psychological. He was nervous! When he'd talked to the staff about it, they recommended he come see me instead. I don't actually wear a white coat, and I've been told I'm far more approachable than the average MD. I'm happy to report that Frank's blood pressure was perfectly normal when we took it that day. He was tickled, as was I.

We talked for a while, and Frank told me that he was originally from the Bronx, and that he'd had an interesting series of careers including installing drywall (right around the time it was first invented!), and working on a tuna boat in Alaska. He eventually had gotten married and had three children, but his wife became a closet gambler for twenty-five years. Then his father had fallen ill, and Frank had cared for him for six long years. He remembered it as a very tumultuous time, and he even recalled having been suicidal at one point.

After he separated from his wife and his father passed away, Frank slowly began to get his life back. He started taking his health more seriously, eating right and exercising regularly. When I asked him about his typical breakfast, he told me he has oatmeal and berries when he wakes up, and then makes a smoothie every day at 11 a.m.—with kale, whey protein, fruit, and yogurt. I mean, what ninety-four-year-old do you know who's making kale smoothies? He said he eats meat only "from time to time," but he does enjoy fish. Oh, and he drinks plenty of water throughout the day. (He even showed off his stainless steel water bottle he takes with him everywhere he goes.) He still drives, and he lives completely independently. Throughout the whole conversation, Frank was smiling so much and had such a calm, relaxed way about him that I finally had to ask, "How do you stay so upbeat? I have many elderly patients who struggle with that." His reply blew me away.

"I go to a group every week, and we only talk about positive things in our lives. We leave negativity at the door and only discuss the things we have to be thankful for, and good things happening in the world. You'd be surprised—there's a lot to talk about!" What a wonderful thing—the power of positivity. It's so easy to slip into negative thought patterns, and to focus our energies on what's going wrong instead of what's going right. But Frank isn't going to fall for that; he knows he feels better if he focuses on the good, so that's what he does. And he probably didn't know this when he started that habit, but there's even scientific evidence that optimism can increase longevity.[1] Intentional positivity can, indeed, help increase your lifespan. I think it's definitely working for my new patient hero.

When Frank left that day, I felt lighter and more positive myself. Who knew? It turns out positivity is contagious! I wanted to tell you his story because he is the living embodiment of the more of the good, less of the bad philosophy—from what he eats to how he thinks. I think we should all aim to be a little more like Frank.

As you take more steps in the direction of weight loss and good health, I encourage you to also try to find things along the way to be grateful for. In fact, make that part of your daily journaling exercise. Simply answer the question, "What am I grateful for today?" Or, like Frank, you could just write down one thing that's positive in the world, or in your life. Feeling gratitude has powerful effects on the mind, and thus on our bodies. Even on days when it feels like everything is just going sideways, there's always something for which you can feel grateful. See if you can find it and focus on it even for a few moments. It could be the thing that turns your whole day around.

5

THE 10-DAY "STABILIZE"

You are one week into this journey—yes! Your body is now a high-performance sponge, absorbing at max capacity. The heavier it is to start with, the more dramatic the difference when wringing it out. This process is now repeating itself daily—taking in more of the good, and storing less of the bad. Look at you.

Let's take a moment to think about the changes you're already feeling. Patients often tell me one of the most surprising side effects is that they feel truly satisfied after eating meals without any meat. Especially for people who are used to eating meat three or four times a day, that's a big deal. Remember, this is a whole-food, "plant-forward" plan, not a fully "plant-based" plan. In my experience, I'd say about 5 percent of people can consistently follow a fully plant-based lifestyle, so I am writing this book for the other 95 percent of us.

Another comment I often hear after the first week is that folks notice they're craving foods they would never even have thought about before. Instead of looking forward to ice cream or cake, they get excited about a bowl of berries. These kinds of things begin happening because your body is transforming, and that includes your brain. It's getting rewired to desire foods that taste great and nourish you on a cellular level.

There are several other changes that are likely occurring as well. Your clothes should be fitting more loosely, and your energy levels skyrocketing. You are probably sleeping better than you were before, and feeling more productive both at work and at home because you're thinking more clearly. I hope you're feeling pleased with the progress you see and feel . . . and just seven days into it. I've found that one of the biggest keys to losing weight and keeping it off is confidence. Believing in what you're capable of achieving is critical, and as you see yourself succeeding, your confidence will soar. And it's only going to get better and better from here.

Take a moment and check off the items on this list that apply to you:

- ❑ I have started losing weight
- ❑ I'm craving healthier foods like vegetables
- ❑ My energy is improving
- ❑ I'm sleeping better and for longer
- ❑ My overall mood is better
- ❑ My stomach is flatter
- ❑ My skin looks healthier
- ❑ People have started to notice something different about me
- ❑ My clothes fit more comfortably

In this phase, you'll have a wider variety of foods and recipes to choose from as your body really settles into the new healthy habits you've created. You'll still be able to eat all the foods from the Scrub and Soak Up food lists, so if you have some go-to meals or snacks, you can absolutely still go to them. The reason I dubbed this phase "Stabilize" is that it is designed to help you stabilize your health and lifestyle as well as your eating habits. As we've discussed, a diet is no good if you can't stick with it, and these ten days will help you realize this is *so* something you can do for the rest of your life.

STABILIZE FOODS

You'll get to enjoy even more foods in this phase, and that includes everything from the previous two phases. Allow yourself to ponder all the delicious combinations you could create from these ingredients. You might have a few flops, but I bet you'll discover a whole lot of showstoppers. I've always believed that healthy eating is fueled by a healthy imagination, so use your noodle. It's fun to think about delicious flavor combinations and to play chef in your own kitchen. Or, if that's simply not your cup of tea, feel free to take advantage of the recipes I'm including later in this book. They're simple, tasty, and tried-and-true.

Reminder: Your "Less of" List

As you continue onward, remember that there are certain foods that are pure kryptonite to anyone trying to detoxify their body, lose weight, and improve their health. (Psst . . . that's you!) In the spirit of this new take on creating a healthy lifestyle, I'll never say "never," but at least for now, I highly recommend you continue to limit your intake of the following:

- Fast food (anything from a drive-thru qualifies)
- Fried foods (this includes anything prepared as "tempura" or "breaded")
- White-flour foods (white pastas, breads, white crackers)
  - *Note:* Whole wheat and whole grains are naturally full of germ and bran fiber, as well as being vitamin- and mineral-dense. But the process of refining whole wheat into white flour removes almost all of the fiber and most of the naturally occurring vitamins and minerals, which then are often "enriched" back in. Once void of fiber, white flour causes our blood sugar to rise rapidly, leading to prediabetes, weight gain, and probably impacts on our mood and energy.
- Milk, cream
- Excessive caffeine (more than 200 mg per day, or about two cups of coffee)
- Alcohol (more on this topic later in the chapter)

- All sugars (check ingredients for sugar "code words" such as dextrose, maltodextrin, date sugar, fructose, glucose, sucrose, lactose, ethyl maltol, etc.)

Stabilize Foods List

Note: You can eat all of the foods from the 3-Day Scrub and 4-Day Soak Up food lists.

- All vegetables, including starchy vegetables
  - You score extra credit for: leafy greens, artichoke, jicama, sweet potatoes
- Whole cooked grains such as oats, bulgur, brown rice, barley, farro, buckwheat (these are all great prebiotic foods)
- Whole grain breads like whole wheat pita, whole wheat tortilla, sprouted whole wheat or multigrain bread, 100% whole rye, Bavarian rye, fermented sourdough bread
- Whole grain pasta such as quinoa pasta, whole wheat pasta, lentil pasta
- Gluten-free breads and tortillas
- All fruits, with an emphasis on low-sugar fruits such as:
  - Apples
  - Berries
  - Grapefruit
  - Oranges
  - Peaches
  - Pears
  - Plums
  - Prickly pear cactus
  - Prunes
  - Red grapes
- All nuts*
- All seeds*
- Beans, lentils
- Kombucha

- One serving should not exceed 12 grams of sugar—the lower, the better, of course, because not only is there less sugar but there is also more probiotic content. Most bottles of kombucha can easily be separated into two servings.
- Nut butters, preferably organic (1 tablespoon = 1 serving)
- Fish, with an emphasis on wild-caught salmon and sardines
- Shellfish**
- Eggs (limit to 6 total eggs per week)
- Poultry
- Beef, pork, lamb (1 serving = 4 to 6 ounces)
- Cooking oils (olive, avocado, coconut, butter, ghee)
- Green tea (or one cup of coffee or black tea a day if preferred)
- All spices and herbs, with an emphasis on cinnamon, ginger, turmeric, thyme, oregano
- Natural sweeteners (no more than 2 teaspoons per serving):
  - Raw honey
  - Maple syrup
  - Coconut sugar
  - Coconut syrup
- Specific dairy foods:
  - Yogurt (1 serving = 6 ounces)—preferably organic, whole-fat (not skim, which usually has more sugar content). You can also try nut-based yogurts, and sheep or goat milk yogurt.
    - Greek yogurt is optimal. Avoid sweetened yogurts; if you do have them (or any packaged food), stay under 12 grams of sugar per serving. The best way to sweeten yogurt is to add fresh fruit (such as mashed-up berries) or 1 teaspoon maple syrup (only about 4 grams of sugar, and it takes only this much to enhance sweetness).
  - Kefir (1 serving = 4 ounces)—preferably organic, unflavored (since flavored varieties have more sugar)

- Butter (grass-fed)
- Ghee, preferably organic
- Some cheeses—see sidebar on page 71. (1 serving = 1 ounce, equivalent to 1 thin slice or 2 small cubes, about the size of a pair of dice)

* Choose unsalted nuts and seeds, to avoid excess sodium. And if you can get raw, sprouted seeds, that's ideal for the nutritional profile.

** Shellfish such as lobster and crab are often served at restaurants with copious amounts of butter, so if you're eating out, ask for your shellfish without butter for dipping. It's delicious enough on its own! (Or with a cilantro pesto, perhaps!)

H$_2$-OH-YEAH!

Not to be a nag, but are you drinking plenty of water? I ask every single patient who walks in the door of my practice that very question, no matter what the reason for their visit. And do you know what the answer is about 80 percent of the time? "Not as much as I should." Is that your answer today? Well, then, grab a glass and get drinking. Water is the number-one ingredient in this entire diet. We can all use a reminder, too, so consider this yours.

FOR THE CARNIVORES AMONG US

I had a rough day the other day. You know the kind—where it seems like nothing goes right, and the day feels like it will never come to an end. I had been trending toward eating less meat on a regular basis, but that night, I knew that nothing would bring me more joy than a little 4-ounce filet. So, without any hesitation at all, I grilled one up. To go with it, I made a huge salad and grilled some asparagus and snap peas, and my plate ended up being about 80 percent vegetables; it was most assuredly a plant-forward plate. I ate and enjoyed every single bite. And by the time I was done, I felt much better about the day because I was physically satiated.

Why am I sharing what I ate for dinner with you? To remind you that if you are a meat lover, a carnivore through and through, I am not saying you need to give it up completely. But when you do cut back on how much and how often you eat meat, you'll likely discover you enjoy it even more when you do have some. It's pretty amazing how that works. So, pat yourself on the back whenever you manage a meal without meat, and when you do enjoy a little, you can feel just fine about it. No side dishes of guilt on this plan!

Cut the Cheese?

If you've ever sat down to a bowl of queso at a Mexican restaurant, or passed by the cheese tray a couple dozen times at a party, then you're probably familiar with an undeniable truth. Once you start eating cheese, it is *really* tough to pump the brakes. That's why I always hesitate before including cheese in a food list; it's just too easy to overdo it. Now, are there health benefits to some cheeses? Sure. A few. Depending on which variety we're talking about, there's calcium and protein, and the fat content can help with satiety. But you have to be choosy with your cheese, and stingy too.

If you do decide to enjoy some cheese here and there, keep these tips in mind. First and foremost, make sure it's real cheese, and not some abomination of chemical processing called "cheese product." Second, hard, fermented cheeses like Parmesan, cheddar, and Swiss tend to be easier to digest than soft cheeses such as brie, because they have less lactose. Blue cheese, if that's your thing, is very high in calcium, and because the flavor is so distinctive, we typically eat less of it at one sitting. Those are some good bets if you're rolling the dice on cheese.

Another tip when you're eating cheese is to fill your plate with other healthy options so you actually don't need or want more than a serving of cheese. Add in some nuts, fresh berries, or a whole wheat cracker, or top an arugula salad with some shredded Parmesan. Then, when you look at the meal as a whole, you can clearly see it comprises more of the good and less of the bad.

There's really no need to cut cheese out of your diet forever, but do be aware of the quality and make it a goal to keep your portions small when you do add it to a meal or snack.

PLAN IT OUT

The easiest way to make sure you're eating more of the good foods your body needs and not constantly being waylaid by every temptation is to plan what you're going to eat in advance of each meal. I know you might be rolling your eyes because it seems time-consuming. But once you get the hang of it, I promise that planning meals ahead actually saves you time in the long run. When it comes to managing our time, the more things that we can automate—meaning program in advance—the more free time we end up having in our day.

Schedule your grocery shopping or delivery to occur on the same day each week, and get all of the items you need to create meals for that week. This allows you to handle it all at once, rather than running out to the grocery store every couple of days to get new ingredients. Then, as you're putting groceries away, spend a few minutes preparing the ingredients that need chopping, slicing, or dicing, or the ones that can be cooked ahead of time like whole grains. You can even portion them out into separate containers. (Helpful tip: I always recommend using glass or stainless steel containers, to avoid any risk of plastic contaminants.)

I bring my lunch with me to work almost every day, which keeps me from having to spend time deciding what to eat. That gives me more time to take care of personal items on my list, or even to sneak in a lunch-break workout. It takes all the decision-making out of the equation—and in our busy lives, one less thing to think about makes a big difference.

I also use a meal delivery service that delivers fresh, fully prepared meals to my doorstep on a regular basis. Because the demand for this has grown exponentially over recent years, the cost of this kind of service has really gone down. Especially if preparing meals ahead of time is something you struggle with, this can be a great option that I'd highly recommend. Do a little research online and you can easily find one that delivers fresh, healthy meals that are already portioned out so that all you have to do is heat them up. And you can order however many meals you'd like—maybe you just need a couple a week, or maybe you need a couple a day. It's up to you.

If your work or lifestyle involves a lot of travel, planning out your food ahead of time can help you tremendously. I can't tell you how many times I've been about to board an airplane and suddenly realized I was starving. These days, you never know if there will even be any food available on a plane, but you can pretty much bet there won't be many healthy options. So, when packing for a trip—whether it's just a couple hours in the car, or a few days that you'll be away—plan the nutrient-dense and great-tasting snacks you can carry with you.

This is a great opportunity to work in things like nuts, seeds, a couple apples, grapes, oranges, baby carrots, and other travel-friendly fruits or veggies. Or spread some almond butter on a whole grain tortilla with a drizzle of honey, roll it up, and stick it in a sandwich bag—the perfect snack for later. You could even throw together a veggie wrap using a whole grain pita, some cucumbers, jicama (which is something I grew up eating all the time—my dad would put thin strips of it in water to keep it moist), tomatoes, basil, even some avocado spread on it—you get the idea. The possibilities are endless; all it requires is a little bit of planning and ingenuity. And instead of coming home feeling swollen, bloated, and guilty, you can feel bright, light, and proud of yourself.

NAVIGATING RESTAURANTS

Let's face it, there are weeks when we eat out or order in restaurant food more often than we make our own meals. But does that mean you have to order the greasiest, carb-iest items on the menu? No! You can stick to this plan and still eat out at restaurants. Here are some tips to help:

- **Decide in advance:** Check out the menu online before you go, and make your choice long before you're seated at the table, drooling over every option.

- **Sit somewhere quiet:** The fewer distractions you have going on around you, the more you can focus on enjoying each bite, and notice when you're starting to feel full so you don't overindulge.

- **Order first:** Before anyone else in your party can set the tone toward french fries and cheeseburgers, order your plant-forward meal first so you aren't tempted to change your mind.

- **Make yours special:** Just because the menu says a meal is prepared a certain way doesn't mean you can't ask for changes. Request steamed vegetables rather than sautéed in butter. Or baked chicken instead of fried. They may not be able to make every accommodation, but it can't hurt to ask.

- **Skip the apps:** If one of the appetizers on the menu sounds amazing to you, go ahead and order it—but make it your entire meal. If you order the app and a main course, you run the risk of overeating. By eating it as your main meal (and maybe adding a side salad), you get to enjoy the dish, but not overindulge.

- **Choose your salad wisely:** Salads can be a great, veggie-packed choice for a meal. But just watch out for all the "extras" like cheese, dressings loaded with sugar and fat, bacon, croutons, and more. Read through all of the ingredients, and then ask the server to exclude ones you don't want. And a safe bet for dressing is always olive oil and vinegar.

- **Don't drink your dinner:** If you're going to have alcohol with dinner, limit yourself to one drink. That means 5 ounces of wine, 1.5 ounces of liquor, or 12 ounces of light beer. Better yet, wait until you get home and, if you still want the drink, have it then.

- **Practice small portions:** Ask in advance how large the portion is for the meal, and if it's big, ask the server to box up half of it and serve the rest. That way, you aren't tempted to eat the whole thing and then wish you'd worn your stretchy pants.

- **Redefine dessert:** If you're wanting a taste of something sweet after the meal, find out if the restaurant offers fruit or just a small bowl of berries. That can satisfy your sweet tooth without throwing a wrench in the gears. If you just can't resist the chocolate lava cake at this particular dining establishment, indulge in three bites and then put your fork down. As long as you're not doing this all the time, the three-bite rule is a smart way to stay on track without always feeling like you're missing out on life's little indulgences.

BUT CAN I HAVE ALCOHOL?

The work you did in the first week of this plan really helped your organ systems to get into the mode of detoxification, and if there's anything that can throw a wrench in those gears, it's alcohol. You see, alcohol has an immediate effect on your liver when you drink it. And your liver is primarily responsible for breaking down toxins in your body. Instead of forcing it to work overtime, cut your liver a break and go these ten days without any wine, beer, or spirits. You might be saying, "No problem, Doc!" or you might be bursting into tears right about now. I get it. I enjoy my wine with dinner. But I also know that if I take breaks from it, I will enjoy it even more when I do sit down to a glass of cabernet. And my liver will thank me too.

So, if alcohol is something that you look forward to (in moderation), it's important that you figure out something to replace it that you will also enjoy. Otherwise you'll just be thinking about how much you're missing your evening cocktail. I've learned from my patients that habits are nearly impossible to break; it's much easier to replace them. Here are some ideas for alcohol swaps:

- Tasty Teas: Try out a variety of herbal teas to see what you like, and add a little honey for some extra sweetness.
  - Green tea is my go-to because of its fat-burning capabilities and because it gives me even energy throughout the day instead of the energy spikes that coffee creates.

- Tea of the Fermented Variety: Reach for a kombucha, which is basically fermented tea with live, active cultures. There are now many flavors available, but be sure to watch out for added artificial sweeteners.
  - Kombucha is loaded with probiotics, electrolytes, polyphenols, and enzymes, all of which can be great for your gut.

- Make a Mocktail: Pour some naturally flavored sparkling water over ice in a highball glass, squeeze some fresh citrus juice (lemon, lime, grapefruit, or orange) over it, give it a quick stir, and add a twist of lime or lemon. Delish!

- Fancy Water: Add some slices of fruit like strawberries, veggies like cucumbers, or even fresh herbs like mint or rosemary to a pitcher of water. Let it sit in the fridge overnight; in the morning, your water will have just a hint of flavor to it. (See a list of water "recipes" in the back of the book for more ideas for dressing up your water.)

- Get Juicy: If you have a juicer (or want to invest in one), try making fresh juice with a mixture of fruits and vegetables. You may not get all the benefits of the fiber from the produce, but the juice itself still packs a nutritional wallop that your body will love. Keep in mind that this only applies to homemade juice or juices that have been cold-pressed and that you drink right away. Store-bought juices are almost always packed with sugar that won't do you any favors, and they're pasteurized to make them shelf-stable, which means many of the key vitamins and minerals are negated.

After these seventeen days are up, if you want to sip on a cocktail, a glass of wine, or a beer, it won't have a huge impact on your weight loss or detoxification, especially if you're continuing to drink plenty of water each day. However, don't overdo it. For the first thirty days of any new diet plan, your liver is already working hard to release toxins formerly stored in your body, so you really want to give it some respect.

What's the bottom line when it comes to your waistline? Alcohol won't ever make you thinner. So if you want to shed pounds, step away from the booze, at least for the time being. But remember, if you're currently consuming three beers with dinner every night, and we can get you down to two, then that's a win. I want you to finish this race with a smile on your face, not feeling completely deprived and miserable. You are in control here, and if losing weight quickly is a huge priority for you, then cutting back on alcohol may not feel like too big of a sacrifice. It's all a trade-off. I just want you to celebrate your wins along the way, and realize that you are making progress.

KEEP ON M&M'ING

How is your M&M practice going? Are you being more mindful about your decisions each day? And remembering your motivation for this whole-life transformation that you're creating? If you're anything like me, a few reminders along the way can help a lot. How easily we forget from day to day, or even hour to hour. That's one of the many reasons why I believe in developing a great support system, so that people in your life can remind you of your goals. We'll delve deeper into that topic in the next chapter, but for now, think of me as the Robin to your

Batman. I'm your helpful sidekick, here to support you through the tough moments, and cheer you on through the victories.

Every morning when you wake up, remind yourself of your motivations as soon as you open your eyes. It doesn't have to take any more than ten seconds to think about your reasons for living longer and feeling your best. Even a few seconds of reconnecting with those internal motivations will set the tone for the entire day and help you keep your feet firmly on this new path. You can do this. Actually, considering the progress you've already made, I'll revise that and say—you're already doing this!

Curve balls will come, as they do. That's just part of life. As I've shared with you, I've been thrown a few in my time. But having this firm foundation underneath me, this way of eating, moving, and living that is now programmed into my daily routine, has helped me so much anytime life gets crazy. I think you'll find the same thing to be true for you.

WHAT'S NEXT?

After you've completed this 10-Day Stabilize phase, here are my recommendations for your next steps:

- If you still have twenty-plus pounds to lose, you can return to Scrub and begin the seventeen-day program again.

- If you have ten to twenty pounds more to lose, you can toggle between Soak Up and Stabilize until you've reached your desired weight loss.

- If you have ten or fewer pounds to lose, you can repeat the Stabilize phase until you've reached your goal weight.

The Stabilize phase of this diet plan is really designed to be a lifelong nutritional program. You can use it to maintain your weight and to continuously improve your health. But anytime you feel yourself gaining weight for whatever reason, you can always start up again with Scrub. Personally, I like to do that several times a year so I can reset when I need it. Then I pretty much stay on Stabilize the rest of the time.

Now that you have a handle on which foods will fuel your body, let's turn our attention to how you can burn off some of that fuel—with healthy movement.

6

LET'S GET MOVING

We are meant to move. Our bodies were designed to be in motion. But, sadly, it seems that the more technological advances we make, the less reason we have to move. Think of all the things we can do—communicate with someone on the other side of the world, drive a car, fly in an airplane, pay bills, order anything we could possibly want or need—all while sitting down. These innovations are astonishing. And the number of hours we spend in the seated position in a twenty-four-hour day is also astonishing. But here's the bottom line: regular movement is required for good health, so I want to help you get moving more and sitting on your behind less.

From a physiological standpoint, exercise improves circulation, which is critical for immunity, functionality, and strength. It also helps you build muscle. Have you heard of sarcopenia? It is the natural decrease in muscle mass we all experience, and it starts at age thirty. That's right; muscle mass decreases approximately 3 to 8 percent per decade after age thirty, and it begins to decrease even more rapidly after the age of sixty. As our muscle mass, strength, and function go down, our risk of disability goes up. Sarcopenia increases our risks of falls and injury and, as a result, can then lead to functional dependence and disability.[1] Not a pretty picture. That's why it's so important to do anything we can to build muscle, so that we can maintain our functionality as we age. Strong muscles help protect our joints and spine, and they also help us burn fat.

Furthermore, there is research indicating that regular exercise can help protect the health of our brain. In fact, one study looked at patients with mild Alzheimer's and found that moderate aerobic activity can improve their cognitive function.[2] That's pretty compelling, if you ask me.

As we talked about earlier, nonalcoholic fatty liver (NAFL) is a dangerous condition that is on the rise in America, but there is lots of exciting research indicating that exercise can have a positive effect on that too. Regular exercise has become a first-line therapy for patients with NAFL. One study looked at both aerobic and resistance exercise and discovered that both forms can reduce the effects with similar frequency and duration of exercise (forty to forty-five minutes per session, three times a week for twelve weeks). So for those patients who struggle with aerobic exercise, where your heart rate is increased and you are perspiring, doctors are recommending resistance exercise because it may be more feasible.[3] This may apply to you too—if aerobic exercise, or "cardio," is too challenging as a starting point, resistance training is a great alternative.

I do want to make an important distinction concerning the type of movement we'll be discussing in this chapter. It's something I refer to as purposeless movement—in other words, exercise strictly for the sake of exercise. It is not the walking around you do while you're at work. It is not zooming from the laundry room to the closets putting clothes away. And it is not strolling around the mall or grocery store while you're shopping. All of those things are great, and your body will thank you for all forms of movement, but what I want you to incorporate into your lifestyle is purposeless exercise, where your mind is not focused on your work, errands, or chores but on engaging your full body in movement.

I have several patients who own retail shops, and they often say, "Doc, I don't sit down all day other than to eat lunch. I'm constantly walking around the store, and by the end of the day, I'm exhausted. Surely that's enough exercise?" But then I ask, "Great, but where is your mind when you're doing all that moving around?" The answer is always—on their work. As it should be! When we're on the job, we need our minds to be fully engaged with the tasks at hand. Take construction workers: when you think about what they're doing all day long, it's very physical. But it's also mentally very challenging; they are thinking on their feet, making important decisions. So that's not purposeless exercise either.

Why is it so important to exercise without being mentally engaged in anything else? You see, a key benefit of exercise is the mental reset it provides. There's a component of meditation, mental relaxation, and decompression. Returning to the sponge analogy I shared with you earlier, exercise allows you to wring out your mental sponge. That sponge just gets so full of stuff all day long, from the moment we open our eyes. Think about what happens when a kitchen sponge gets too full—it stops working! You have to wring it out in order for it to keep being functional. That's what purposeless exercise does for your mind. While you're getting your heart rate up doing the form of exercise you like to do, your mind is able to just wander aimlessly, and not go in any particular or focused direction. We need that a lot more than we realize. It's extremely satisfying.

I'm so passionate about the topic of movement that I ask every patient I see about their current exercise routine, regardless of why they came in. Very often, people tell me about all the walking around they do in everyday life, and I tell them the same thing I'm telling you—that's great, but it's not purposeless exercise. Then we do a role reversal. They play doctor and ask me about my exercise. My answer is, "I swim thirty minutes every day except I take Sundays off." Then I ask the patient if he or she notices the difference between their answer and mine. My routine is simple and straightforward. It doesn't have to be complicated, expensive, or super time-consuming. But we do have to create room for it in our lives. Is it a good idea to park far away from the entrance of the movie theater and walking those extra steps? Sure. But you need to fit in purposeless exercise too.

When creating a routine like this, it really helps to know exactly where you are starting. What are you capable of doing before you have to take a rest? Knowing that the magic number is 30—meaning you want to fit in a minimum of 30 minutes of exercise every day—you can easily figure out an exercise routine that will get you to that number. So let's say you are capable of walking for 5 minutes before you need to take a rest. In that case, you divide 30 by 5, and that means you need to walk for 5 minutes 6 times throughout the day (5 x 6 = 30). Or, if you can exercise for 10 minutes without taking a rest, then you need to find 3 times during the day that you can exercise for 10 minutes at a time (3 x 10 = 30). In other words, don't get overwhelmed thinking about having to complete 30 straight minutes of exercise all at the same time. It's additive throughout the day. This can make it feel so much more achievable.

Here's the simple formula written out so you can create your own realistic routine:

My 30-Minute Plan

I can exercise for _____(x) minutes before taking a break.

$$\frac{30}{x} = y$$

So, I will exercise for _____ (x) minutes _____ (y) times per day to reach my 30-minute minimum.

TURNING "I CAN'T" INTO "I CAN"

In a lot of the conversations I have with my patients about exercise, they love to tell me what they *can't* do. They explain that certain exercises hurt certain joints or parts of their body. It's really easy to think of the things we can't do; I get it. And there are things I can't do that I miss too. But instead of giving up, I encourage them to get creative. You know all the things you can't do, so rule those things out, and then think about the things you *can* do.

In fact, why don't you give it a try? Write down the first things that come to mind when you think about exercise, in terms of what you feel you are not able to do. Then apply some creativity, and come up with a few examples of things you *can* do. For example, if you have a sore shoulder and you feel you can't do most upper-body exercises, what are some lower-body exercises you can do while your shoulder heals?

The point is, I don't want you to let an injury or inflammation in one part of the body keep you from being able to exercise at all. So, give it a try!

I can't . . . _____

But I can . . . _____

I can't . . . _____

But I can . . . _____

I can't . . . _____

But I can . . . _____

I can't . . . _____

But I can . . . _____

Need some "I can" ideas for your list? Here are just a few examples:

- Climbing stairs briskly (take two at a time for an extra challenge)
- Box jumps (these can be curb or step jumps too)
- Dancing (in a studio or in your living room)
- Jumping jacks
- Jumping rope (the rope can be invisible)
- Online workouts (there are endless options)
- Hula-hooping
- Power walking
- Jogging
- Running

- Elliptical cross-training
- Rowing (on a rowing machine or out in the water if that's an option where you live)
- Biking (spin bike or outdoor bicycle)
- Martial arts (including shadowboxing)
- Swimming (this is my go-to for no-impact exercise)
- Weight lifting (I'll get into specifics later in the chapter)
- Resistance training using body weight
- Lunges
- Squats
- Squat jumps
  - This is a squat but with a jump when you switch legs.
- Crab walks
  - From standing, place your hands on the floor in front of you, and then walk back and forth on all fours.
- Butt kickers
  - Standing in place, bring your right heel up to your right buttock, then put it back down. Repeat with the other leg. Once you have the hang of it, pick up your speed!
- Burpees
  - From standing, place your hands on the ground in front of your feet, then jump your feet backward so you are in a push-up position. Then jump them back in, stand up, and hop in place. A few of these can really get your heart pumping.
  - The beginner version is to walk your hands out until you're in a push-up position, then walk them back, stand, and hop.

Regardless of how you choose to exercise, I want you to be realistic. For me, if I can swim 1,500 meters, I know I've gotten adequate exercise for the day. But our exercise goals are all very individual. As long as you are aiming for thirty minutes of exercise per day, you can consider yourself to be on the right track.

How do you know if you're exercising hard enough? I like using something I call the "talk test." If you're able to carry on a conversation with ease, you need to step it up. If you're hardly able to form words because you're so winded, it's time to take it down a notch. Easy, right? And don't be afraid to try talking to yourself if you're working out solo.

Remember, the toughest part of any exercise program is the first few minutes. But once you've gotten over that hump, it gets easier. After just the first couple of laps of a swim, I start to feel amazing. I might not have wanted to go down to the pool, and I might have had to fight hard to keep myself from just sinking into the couch or having a glass of wine, but after those initial laps, I'm thanking myself so much for making the commitment. You can feel that way too. Exercise should always be something you look forward to. You hold the power to change how you perceive exercise, so choose to embrace the positive and focus on what you *can* do.

Listen to Your Body

While it is completely normal to experience some general soreness anytime you are starting a new exercise regimen, what isn't normal is a sudden, sharp pain. If, at any time during a workout, you feel a sharp pain, take a break and then assess the situation. Pain is a signal that something might be off, and you don't want to "power through" an injury and end up making it worse. I want you to start becoming more attuned to your body, and that means paying attention to how you're feeling during exercise. A little soreness a couple days after a solid workout is a good thing—it lets you know that your body is changing. But if you're incapacitated or so exhausted the next day that you struggle to get out of bed, you should definitely ease up on the exercise. Try to find that sweet spot where you're pushing yourself but not so hard that you're doing more harm than good.

MOVE TO THE MUSIC

If you need a little motivation and energy boost, just pump up the jams. Research shows that music can have a powerful effect on our ability and desire to exercise. In a *Psychology Today* article, Jeanette Bicknell, a professor of philosophy and the author of *Why Music Moves Us*, said, "When music is used before athletic activity, it has been shown to increase arousal, facilitate relevant imagery, and improve the performance of simple tasks. When music is used during activity, it has ergogenic [work-enhancing] effects and psychological effects. Listening to music during exercise can both delay fatigue and lessen the subjective perception of fatigue. It can increase physical capacity, improve energy efficiency, and influence mood. In study after study, the use of music during low- to moderate-level-intensity exercise was associated with clear improvements in endurance." How about that? It can actually delay and reduce how tired you feel during a workout, so you can torch even more fat.

So, what kind of music moves you? Oldies? Heavy metal? Country? Movie soundtracks? Use your favorite high-energy tunes to keep you motivated, whether you're sweating it out at the gym or breaking out your best dance moves in the living room. Throw a thirty-minute dance party for one (you!) in your living room. That's one that my friends with young kids love to do—and it has the added bonus of wearing out the kids too.

Music can be the deciding factor that gets you up out of your chair and on your feet. So turn up that volume and go for it!

STRONG = SEXY: STRENGTH TRAINING 101

Strength training is one of the best things you can do for your body. It helps protect your joints and prevent injury as you age, it builds lean muscle mass (which burns fat), it improves your overall body composition (fat to muscle ratio), and it just makes you feel amazing. But don't worry—you don't have to join a fancy, expensive gym in order to build your strength. There are plenty of ways to build muscle using your own body weight or objects around the house.

If you're relatively new to strength training, or you want to get back into a routine but you're not sure where to start, I've compiled a list of moves you can start doing today. Be sure to focus on your form with each of these moves, not only to keep from hurting yourself, but to get the maximum benefits from them. If you find yourself unable to maintain good form, try reducing the number of repetitions.

What's the Scoop on Sweat?

To sweat or not to sweat, that is the question. Here's the deal. The better shape you're in, the more likely you are to work up a sweat very quickly during a workout. Sweating is one of your body's amazing ways of cooling you off and detoxifying you. If you don't sweat easily, that's okay. Don't push yourself into oblivion just for a few beads of sweat. But as you get more into moving and grooving, you'll start sweating more. Try doing something active you loved as a kid. Break out the Hula-Hoop, visit a trampoline park (or an in-home rebounder), play hopscotch or jump rope. Sometimes letting our inner child out for some play is a great way to work up a healthy sweat.

Core (Abdominal) Exercises

Crunches: Get into a sit-up position with knees bent, feet flat on the floor, and your arms crossed over your chest. Breathe out as you pull your belly button toward your spine, using your core to pull your upper body toward your knees. Keep your eyes focused on one point on the ceiling the entire time, with your neck long. Inhale as you lower your back toward the ground without letting your head touch the floor. Repeat 25 times.

Planks: Get into a push-up position, but on your forearms instead of hands, with legs straight and only your toes touching the ground.

Hold your body flat. Do not sag or arch your back. Hold for thirty to sixty seconds.

Side Twists: Sit on the floor with your legs straight out and cross your arms over your chest. (If you have a hard floor, sit on a towel or blanket to protect your tailbone.) Lean back so your upper body makes a 45-degree angle to the floor. Rotate your torso to the right while bringing your right knee toward your chest. Your left elbow should be touching your right knee. Return to starting position. Now rotate your torso to the left as you bring your left knee toward your chest. Repeat 10 times on each side.

Bicycles: Lie on your back on the floor. Lightly place your hands behind your head, but keep your neck extended with your eyes on the ceiling. Bring your legs and upper body to a 45-degree angle. Mimic a pedaling motion with your legs in the air, pulling your belly button toward your spine at all times. Your abs and thighs should burn throughout this exercise. Pedal 25 times.

Balance Exercises

Heel-Toe Walk: Walk heel to toe along an imaginary straight line while focusing your gaze on something in front of you; do not look at your feet. Continue for one minute.

Stork Stance/Tree Pose: While standing barefoot, lift one leg off the ground and position the foot against the inside of the standing thigh or calf. The beginner version is to just barely lift your foot off the ground. To help with balance, fix your eyes on something in front of you. Engage your core muscles to stay still. Try closing your eyes. Hold each side for thirty seconds.

Weight Shifts: Stand with feet hip width apart. Slowly lift one leg sideways so your foot is off the floor and your toes are pointed as you shift your weight to the opposite side. Hold for thirty seconds, then switch legs.

Ball around Back: Stand on one leg while holding a ball. Circle the ball behind your back and around your waist while keeping your balance. Also try with your eyes closed.

Dynamic Stretches

Toy Soldiers: If your hamstrings are tight, take this slowly at first. Standing up straight, and holding on to furniture for support if you need it, kick your leg out straight in front of you and use the opposite hand to touch your toe at the same time. Alternate between legs, and repeat 10 times on each side. This can really help to keep your hamstrings from getting too tight, which can lead to back pain and discomfort. This is a great move to do before any workout routine.

Toe Touches: Take a step forward with one foot, and reach down and touch the toe with the opposite hand. Work to keep only a slight bend in the front leg. Straighten up, and alternate sides. Repeat 10 times. This stretches your hamstrings and lower back. It's also a great dynamic stretch to complete before a workout routine, as it can help prevent injury.

Cat-Cow: Get on all fours on the floor, or on a yoga mat, exercise pad, or towel. Gently arch your back like a cat and drop your head forward while you inhale, then drop your belly as you raise your head and look toward the sky and exhale. This is fantastic for spinal flexibility. Repeat 12 times.

Hip Hinges: Standing tall with your feet hip width apart, place your hands behind your head. Keeping your back completely straight, bend at the waist while thrusting your glutes straight back like they're trying to touch the wall behind you. Get to about 90 degrees, or as far as you can go while keeping your back straight, and then stand back up. Repeat 12 times. Think about your hamstrings during this exercise too.

Strength Exercises for Push Muscles

Your push muscles are triceps, chest, and shoulders. It's important to keep these muscles healthy because they help with good posture, and with preventing injuries associated with aging, such as to the rotator cuff.

Push-Ups: On the floor with legs straight out behind you, form a straight board with your body. The beginner version is to keep your knees on the floor (instead of toes), but on a folded towel or pad to give them some cushion. Keep your elbows extended and hands shoulder width apart or wider. Narrow your arms to work triceps more, or widen them to work your chest and shoulders more. Slowly lower your body toward the floor by bending your elbows until your chest is parallel to the ground. Just go as far as you can, but not so far that you can't get back up. Then push your body back up by re-extending your elbows. Do 10 repetitions per set.

T Push-Ups: This is a normal push-up, but as you go back up, twist your body, rotate your hips open and point one arm toward the sky, then return to the push-up position. Repeat on the other side. Alternate arms every time you lift your body up. Do 10 repetitions per set. (Note: If you have pain in either shoulder, skip this move.)

Wall Push-Ups: If push-ups on the ground are too difficult for you to start with, try doing push-ups against the wall first. Face the wall at arm's length, put your hands flat against it, and slowly bend your elbows until your nose almost touches the wall, then return to the starting position. Perform 10 repetitions per set.

Triceps Dips: Sit on a sturdy chair with your legs together, stretched straight out in front of you, or slightly bent. Grip your hands on the edge of the seat and scoot forward, so your butt is off the chair and your arms are supporting your body. Straighten your arms with a little bend to ensure you're working your triceps and not hurting your elbow joints. Slowly lower your body by bending your elbows until your butt is almost touching the ground, then lift your body up. Repeat 10 times for one set.

Strength Exercises for Pull Muscles
Your pull muscles are your upper back, biceps, and deltoids.

Bicep Curls: Holding a 5- to 10-pound weight in each hand (start with cans or water bottles if you don't have weights), bend your arms at the elbow, slowly bringing the weights up to your shoulders. Your elbows should stay stationary. Repeat 12 times for one set.

Shrugs: While standing, hold a 5- to 10-pound weight in each hand (or more, for extra challenge), and pull your shoulders up toward your ears, then release back down gently. Repeat 12 times for one set.

Bent-Over Row: Hold a 5- to 10-pound weight—or use cans or water bottles—in each hand. Bend at the waist while keeping your back flat and straight. Bend your elbows and pull them back alongside your body, until your hands are near your armpits, and then slowly straighten the arms back down. Repeat 12 times.

Leg and Glute Strength Exercises

Squats: Carefully monitor your form during all squats, and make sure your knees never extend beyond your toes. Keeping your back straight and your head and chest up, slowly bend at the knees, either until your glutes touch a chair behind you, or until your thighs are at a 90-degree angle. Then slowly stand back up. Concentrate on your glutes and thighs as you lower and stand up, and squeeze your glutes at the top of the movement. Repeat 12 times.

Lunges: You can use a chair or table for stability during this move, but try to hold on to it very lightly. Step forward with one leg, and then slowly bend the back knee toward the ground, until it's one or two inches above the floor. Imagine your knee going straight down. Keep your posture straight and your head up. Then slowly straighten your back leg and return to standing position. Repeat 12 times on each side. Think about your thighs and glutes during the entire exercise.

Deadlifts: Start by standing with your legs hip width apart, holding a light weight in each hand at your sides. Then, as you bend forward, bring the weights in front of you, down to about mid shin. Keep your neck straight (eyes follow your movement) and your back flat the entire way down, with only a slight bend in your legs. If your back begins to curve, don't go any further down. Then, slowly stand back up, with the weights by your sides. Repeat 12 times.

Bridges: Lie on your back, with your knees up and your feet about hip width apart. Then slowly lift your hips and torso off the ground using your glute muscles, keeping your feet flat on the floor. At the top, give your glutes an extra squeeze, hold for five seconds, and then slowly return your torso and back to the ground. Repeat 12 times.

Remember, if these recommendations aren't sparking your interest, there are literally thousands of variations you can do. So don't limit yourself. Many apps and websites are dedicated to this purpose, so there is really no excuse for not working more of these moves into your life. Plus, I think you'll love how much they help you lose weight, tone up, and lose inches.

What's Age Got to Do with It?

If you're currently in your twenties, thirties, or forties and able-bodied, I want you to think of your body as a Ferrari. Now, if you were driving a Ferrari around all day, you wouldn't just drive in the school zones, right? No, you'd take it out on the open road and really let it do its thing. That's how you should view your exercise. A stroll around the block simply isn't enough. You're not doing your body justice if you aren't pushing yourself a little. Get that heart pumping! Work in some interval training, where you're going all-out for two minutes, then slower for one minute, back and forth. The best way to maintain that youthful, vital feeling is to exercise consistently. You've got to use it or lose it!

I've found that if you make exercise part of your daily schedule, just like anything else important you need to do, you'll be much more likely to get your thirty minutes in. Write it in your calendar, or on your daily to-do list. Make an appointment with yourself. Do whatever it takes to program it into your overall schedule. If you make it a priority when you're planning your day or week, you won't have any trouble making it happen.

And here's some great news: exercise is addictive, in a good way. Once your body is used to it, you start to crave it, and it becomes easier. Of course, as with anything, there will be setbacks. There will be busy seasons of life when it's increasingly harder to fit it in. There will be times when you catch a cold and you lose some momentum. But you *can* get back on track. And you'll want to, because you know how good it feels when you're wringing out that mental sponge while giving your body the exercise it needs. So, come on, let's get moving!

7

TO SUPPLEMENT OR
NOT TO SUPPLEMENT?

In case you haven't already noticed, the supplement industry has exploded in the past few years. In fact, Americans spend tens of billions of dollars on supplements each year, and that number saw a drastic increase in 2020, when people became more interested than ever in boosting immunity and staying healthy. Nothing like a pandemic to get people clamoring for vitamins, minerals, probiotics, amino acids, and everything else under the sun. In 2019, nutritional supplement sales were up $345 million over the previous year, and sales growth in 2020 nearly doubled that amount.[1] And this is truly staggering: the global dietary supplements market size was estimated at $123.28 billion in 2019.[2] That's billion with a *b*, folks.

So you might be wondering just how much you should be on that bandwagon, supplementing your diet with pills, powders, liquid vitamins, and more. Here's my opinion on the matter: you should aim to get most of the essential vitamins and minerals your body needs for survival from your food. That is the most "bioavailable" form, meaning the easiest way for your body's organs and tissues to take up and use. Plus, it's the most affordable route. No one wants to take fifty dollars' worth of supplements every single day.

Now, is it always possible to get what your body really needs through the food you're eating? Probably not. The analogy I like to use is sweeping. You know when you're sweeping the floor, and it seems like no matter how hard you try, there's always that thin little line of dirt that you just can't quite sweep into the dustpan? That thin line represents what you're missing in terms of nutrients by focusing on eating healthy foods. You can get really close, but not quite there. Essentially what we're doing with supplements is getting that last bit of nutrition that our bodies need. In other words, don't rely on supplements to be your complete nutrition; they simply serve to get you over the finish line. But there is no point (and even some danger) in going overboard.

The next question you're probably asking is: "Okay, but there's a whole alphabet worth of vitamins—which ones do I really need? Where do I start?" I hear you. It's a lot to decipher. In this chapter, I'll do my best to help you make healthy, affordable decisions on your supplements.

THE WILD WEST

The booming supplement business is the Wild West in a lot of ways. If you've ever read a bottle of vitamins closely, you might have noticed a little line that says, "These statements have not been evaluated by the Food and Drug Administration," or something to that effect. That's right, it's a relatively unregulated business. As a result, you simply cannot assume that every vitamin, mineral, herb, or other supplement on the shelves actually has in it what its label claims. Sad, but true. But there is a way to ensure that what you're taking is what the bottle actually says you're taking, and that's by making sure that they are GMP (Good Manufacturing Practice) certified. They conduct third-party lab tests to ensure that the supplement isn't bogus.

I want you to take only high-quality products, and I want you to take the correct ones. Below is the list I recommend for most people, but—and this is important—*always* discuss vitamins and supplements with your doctor before adding new ones to your routine. Some of these could be contraindicated with certain conditions or medications you're already on, so please take this really seriously.

Supplements I generally recommend are . . .

- A high-quality multivitamin that includes vitamin K and B vitamins (ideally in their "methyl" form)
  - Look for a multivitamin that is a whole food–based formula, rather than synthetic.

Why "Methyl" Form of B Vitamins?

Methylated B vitamins are the active versions of B vitamins that your body can immediately absorb and use, while the unmethylated B vitamins must go through a conversion process before your body can actually utilize them. Additionally, approximately 60 percent of the US population has some kind of genetic variant on a gene called MTHFR, which makes it extremely hard to properly utilize B vitamins that are not methylated. The unmethylated forms often used in supplements do not exist in any living organism, and are exclusively laboratory-manufactured products, whereas methyl B vitamins do exist in nature.

Unmethylated B vitamins are a hundred times cheaper than the natural active methyl B vitamins, which is why they have been the choice for many companies, but that is finally changing as more attention is being put on the importance of taking methylated B vitamins. For everyone, methylated B vitamins will provide more immediate and effective support to energy, cardiovascular health, brain and nervous system function, and fat metabolism!

- Vitamin D_3 (if not already included in your multivitamin)—2,000 IU is a good daily dose if you don't know your levels (ask your health-care provider to do a simple blood test to determine your levels and the best dose accordingly)
- Calcium or a complex bone formula combining calcium, magnesium boron, and other bone-building nutrients that work

together synergistically for bone health support (if directed by your health-care provider)

- Fish oil (look for wild and those that are third-party-tested for heavy metals)
- CoQ10 (as ubiquinol is best)
  - Note: Ubiquinol, the active form of CoQ10, has much greater bioavailability and increases levels about four times over the ubiquinone version of CoQ10. Over the age of thirty, our ability to utilize CoQ10 decreases and we will get more bang for our buck by consuming the most active and bioavailable version, ubiquinol.
- Glucosamine-chondroitin
- Biotin (can cause skin breakouts, so discuss with your doctor if you're concerned)
- Melatonin (as needed for improved sleep, but not to be used on a regular basis)
- Estroven (for women)
- Saw palmetto (for men)
- Red rice yeast (if you have high cholesterol), always taken in combination with CoQ10
- CBD (for more on this, check out chapter 11)
- Cactus juice, as needed for managing glucose levels
  - When I was a kid, my family often prepared cactus in various ways. I didn't learn until much later that it has a positive impact on glucose. Pretty cool!

Spotlight on Quercetin

Since you're now eating a more plant-forward diet, you might be interested to know about some of the specific aspects of vegetables and fruits that are working wonders inside your body. Quercetin is a type of flavonoid, which is an antioxidant phytonutrient found in many common foods like onions, broccoli, apples, berries, and citrus fruits, as well as tea and wine. And it's worth mentioning because numerous studies have indicated that quercetin has powerful anti-inflammatory effects and a positive effect on immunity, and even on histamine production.[3] I predict that researchers will find more and more reasons why we want to be eating as many plant foods as possible. So, eat up and feel better than ever!

PROBIOTICS VS. PREBIOTICS: WHAT'S WHAT?

When it comes to healthy gut bacteria, probiotics have gotten a lot of airtime in the last decade. And for good reason—probiotics are the "good guys" of gut bacteria. (You can find them in yogurt, kefir, kimchi, kombucha, and other fermented foods, as well as in probiotic supplements.) Within your gut microbiome, you have a vast profile of bacteria. Some of those bacteria are considered "good" because they help keep the bad bacteria in check. The bacteria that are considered "bad" can cause all kinds of health problems if left to run wild in your GI tract. And I'm not just talking about your run-of-the-mill bloating and gas, either. Too many of these bad dudes of the bacteria world can lead to irritable bowel syndrome, ulcerative colitis, Crohn's disease, and a host of other issues, none of which are any fun at all.

Because of all the chatter about probiotics out there, a lot of people mistakenly think that they are the one-way ticket for achieving a healthy gut. So they reach for those probiotic supplements that line the pharmacy shelves, or probiotic foods and drinks such as kefir, kombucha, kimchi, and yogurt. That's all wonderful, and I do recommend that you eat plenty of probiotic foods, but they're really only half of the story. You see, if you don't have a good balance already, then all those probiotics you're consuming (and possibly paying a hefty chunk of change for) might just be dying off in your gut. When that happens, it's bye-bye, benefits! So, why is that happening? They aren't getting any food. Yes, you have to first consume, and then *feed* those bacteria.

That's where prebiotics come in. Prebiotics are nondigestible food ingredients that actually help nourish those healthy gut bacteria so they can
grow and flourish. So instead of just dying off, those good guys are able
to multiply. Fiber is a powerful prebiotic. Foods packed with fiber feed
your healthy gut bacteria. The pectin in apples has prebiotic benefits. It
also increases butyrate, a short-chain fatty acid that feeds the beneficial
gut bacteria. Bananas are considered more of a "super prebiotic" because
they contain a small amount of inulin, one of the best prebiotics. Unripe
bananas are also high in "resistant starch," another well-established and
effective form of prebiotic. These are some favorite prebiotics below:

- Dandelion greens
- Chicory root
- Bananas (more green/yellow, less ripe)
- Jicama
- Apples
- Garlic
- Onions
- Leeks
- Asparagus
- Jerusalem artichokes
- Barley
- Oats
- Flaxseeds
- Seaweed

The more of these foods you can work into your daily nutritional
routine, the more balanced your overall gut bacteria will be, and that
means your body can function at its peak.

This whole pro/prebiotic puzzle goes way beyond digestion. Believe
it or not, your immune system resides primarily in your gut. So to help
prevent illness and disease, you want to take steps toward creating a
balanced gut microbiome. And that means eating plenty of both prebiotic foods and probiotic foods.

SLEEP-RELATED SUPPLEMENTS

If you're struggling with your sleep (which is so important that I've devoted the entire next chapter to the subject), you might consider trying some sleep-related supplements.

Melatonin is my go-to for sound sleep. If you haven't heard of it, melatonin is a hormone produced in your brain in response to darkness, essentially telling your body it's time to go to sleep.[4] If you're in a sleep slump, taking a synthetic melatonin supplement may help you fall asleep, but you'll want to discuss it with your doctor before you start using it, just to be sure you don't have any contraindications. I've used it on and off for years with great success, and I know many of my patients have too. But it's not for everyone, so start out with a low dose and see how it goes. Also, as with any supplements you buy, make sure a third-party laboratory has tested it to be sure the label is accurate.

I've also had numerous patients who have experienced radically improved sleep when they've added the right dosage of CBD, either taken as a tincture or used as a topical balm. I go into this topic thoroughly in the "CBD Revolution" chapter, so check that out for more information.

MAKING SENSE OF SUPPLEMENTS

My hope is that you approach supplementation with caution and discernment. There's really no need to go crazy and purchase dozens of bottles of vitamins and minerals, especially if you are following the nutritional advice in this book. And if you know you're low in something because you've had lab work, talk to your doctor about the proper dosage to get your levels back to where they need to be. If you're not sure about your levels, that is something to discuss with your doctor at your next physical. Knowledge is power, and if you know your deficiencies, you can address them. Furthermore, if you notice that you feel better after you begin taking a specific vitamin, then you can use that as a gauge for how well it's working for you. Pay attention to your body's needs, and it will perform better!

8

SLEEP YOURSELF SKINNY

Good sleep can be your secret weapon for weight loss. If you can really dial up your sleep, those pounds will come off so much easier. While you are fast asleep at night, your body is busy losing fat, building muscle, and doing cellular "repair" work via a process called autophagy. Who knew so much was going on while you were dreaming? Sleep is a critical function, and yet we don't tend to value or protect it nearly as much as we should.

On the flip side of the sleep coin, poor sleep can be your Achilles' heel and actually work against your efforts at losing weight.[1] That's right, not getting enough sleep could stall your weight loss even if you are eating all the right foods and exercising regularly. For many people struggling to lose weight, getting their sleep on track is what finally moves the needle.

There is a growing body of research looking at the correlation between sleep and weight or weight-related diseases. Many studies have shown an association between short sleep duration and elevated body mass index (BMI).[2] Researchers have identified insufficient sleep and sleep disorders as important risk factors for the development of diabetes.[3] And there are even studies that have found a link between poor sleep and heart disease.[4]

Moral of the story: it's imperative that you allow your body to get plenty of REM sleep each night. The quality and quantity of your sleep is just as important as the quality and quantity of your food. It plays that vital a role in your body's ability to get to a healthy weight, and then maintain it. You snooze . . . you lose. Get it?

BUT GOOD SLEEP IS TOUGH TO FIND, DOC!

Okay, it's true. These days, there are endless reasons why our sleep gets wrecked. There are so many sleep saboteurs in modern life, depending on our age, health, family circumstances, living quarters, and more. Here are some of the top reasons why sleep might be eluding you:

- **Food, caffeine, or alcohol:** Eating certain foods and consuming caffeine or alcohol particularly later in the day can all have a negative impact on your ability to sleep well.
  - **Tip:** Avoid heavy, fatty foods and alcohol within three hours of bedtime. Stop drinking caffeinated drinks such as tea or coffee by noon if you are sensitive to caffeine.

- **Stress:** There's a reason I've devoted a chapter to stress—it affects all aspects of your life, *especially* your sleep. If you go to bed feeling worried or anxious, your sleep patterns will definitely suffer.
  - **Tip:** Review the advice in chapter 10, "Winning Your Battle with Stress," and make it a daily commitment to not allow stress to run your life or ruin your sleep.

- **Screen time:** Between phones, tablets, laptops, desktops, and televisions, our eyes are glued to some kind of glowing screen all day long. These devices give off short-wavelength enriched light, which you might know as "blue light." And some studies show that blue light can reduce your REM sleep at night.[5]
  - **Tip:** There has been some controversy over how much our exposure to blue light really affects our sleep, but in general, it's a good idea to turn off the screens one hour before bed. And I strongly recommend keeping all electronics out of the bedroom.

- **Children:** Especially if you have a baby or toddler, you might be getting woken up multiple times a night for feedings, diaper changing, or soothing. Brutal on your own sleep!
  - **Tip:** If you're waking up with your child so much during the night that it's affecting your ability to function during the day, have a discussion with your pediatrician or a childhood sleep expert. The Pediatric Sleep Council has a great website with advice, tips, and tricks from the experts. Go to www.babysleep.com to learn more.

- **Snoring or sleep apnea:** Whether it's you or your partner who snores, it can wreak havoc on your good night's rest.
  - **Tip:** Snoring can be a sign of underlying problems, so ask your doctor and also your dentist about it. There are many options for nighttime dental appliances that can help. Sleep apnea (a disorder in which breathing repeatedly stops and starts) is a serious condition not to be taken lightly, so if you suspect you have it, definitely ask your physician.

- **Waking to pee:** Super common. Also super annoying. There's a range of causes, from hormones to anatomical changes to drinking water too late in the day.
  - **Tip:** Try limiting liquids after 5 or 6 p.m. to reduce nighttime urgency. If that doesn't work, have a discussion with your doctor about any underlying cause so you can find an appropriate solution.

- **Poor sleep hygiene:** Anything related to the environment in which you sleep and your nighttime routine—the temperature of your bedroom, the light, bedding, sound—can affect how well you sleep.
  - **Tip:** Once you've read the rest of the chapter to learn what ideal sleep hygiene looks like, examine your own sleep hygiene and make adjustments so you can set yourself up for sleep success.

Are one or all of these issues keeping you from catching enough zzz's and thus derailing your ability to lose weight? In this chapter, I'm going to help you maximize those nighttime hours for weight loss. Because, really, why wouldn't you want to sleep yourself skinny?

The Five Pillars

Earlier in this book, I touched on the five pillars of good health: food, movement, stress management, smoking cessation, and hydration. But here's what I didn't tell you: when you get these five pillars under control, your bonus gift is good sleep. It's essentially a side effect of good health.

Very often when I have a patient complaining of not being able to sleep at night, it's a result of one of these five areas. Maybe the patient smokes. Well, nicotine is a stimulant, so it keeps them up at night. Or perhaps the patient's diet is a mess. The types of foods we eat certainly have an impact on sleep. Dehydration also disrupts sleep, as does lack of purposeless movement. So once we address the specific pillar, that patient suddenly begins to sleep better.

Once in a while, however, I'll come across someone whose health pillars are strong and secure, but they're still struggling with sleep. That's when we start to look at sleep hygiene and routine, or sometimes underlying conditions, and then address those problems. Because the fact is, not sleeping well is a health issue. In a sense, your health may be broken if you don't sleep well. Insomnia can often be a sign or symptom of anxiety or depression. So if you regularly suffer from insomnia, it's certainly worth taking up with your physician.

For the purposes of this chapter, I'm asking you to take a 360-degree look at all of the possible causes for not getting enough sleep at night. It's a little bit of a chicken-or-the-egg scenario because good sleep promotes better health, and better health results in good sleep. So we'll tackle all of the controllable factors, and you'll reap benefits across the board.

WHAT ARE YOUR SLEEP HABITS?

In the quiz you took in chapter 2, there were some questions about the quality and duration of your current sleep, so I hope you've already been thinking about this topic. Right now, let's assess all of your sleep habits so you can see exactly where there is room for improvement.

Fill out these questions:

- Is your bedroom silent at night, or do you use white sound to mask any uncontrollable noises such as traffic outside? _____

- Is your bedroom pitch black at night? _____
    - If not, are there lights you can cover? _____
- What temperature is your bedroom at night? _____
    - Do you wake up feeling too hot or too cold? _____
- What time do you typically go to sleep? _____
- What time do you typically wake up? _____
- How many total hours of sleep are you getting? _____
- How many times do you awake during the night? _____
- Are you waking up to go pee at night? _____
- Do you have trouble going back to sleep when you do wake up at night? _____
- Do you turn off all screens within one hour of going to sleep at night? _____
- Do you have a way of calming yourself and quieting your mind for the half hour before you go to sleep? _____
- How do you feel when you wake up in the morning? Well-rested? Or groggy? _____
- How do you feel in the middle of the day? Wide awake and energized? Or like drifting off to dreamland? _____

I think it's always great to see our habits written in black and white. Otherwise it's too easy to just keep doing what we're doing. If you want to gain some additional insight into your sleep patterns, wearing a sleep tracker can be very informative. When I was going through a bout of sleepless nights (the longest nights in the world), I wore my Fitbit while I slept so I could get real data. When I saw that I was sleeping a total of four and a half hours, even though I'd been in bed for eight, I knew I had to figure something out. Just acknowledging the problem helped me get on the path toward solving it.

For me, that meant first adjusting the meals I ate later in the day. I minimized starchy carbohydrates, alcohol, and anything else that would turn into sugar at night so I wouldn't get energy spikes. I also learned that when I woke up at night, I needed to just get up and read or do something, rather than lie there and obsess about not being able to go to sleep. And that's something I have discussed at length with my patients, because there are definitely activities you want to avoid when you can't sleep—including looking at any kind of screen. Don't jump up and start checking email, scrolling through social media, or bingeing your favorite show. Those activities will only serve to further disrupt your sleep. Instead, read a book (an actual, physical book with pages), fold some laundry, or do something else that's somewhat monotonous. Even some light stretches and breathing exercises are great ideas.

It took time for me to discover the perfect routine, but once I was able to sleep well on a regular basis, I stopped wearing the sleep tracker.

Bedrooms Are for Sleeping

One mistake a lot of people make is to go to sleep in a room other than the bedroom, such as in front of the TV in the living room. This sets up a bad habit and makes it harder to go to sleep at bedtime. It's best to keep the wakeful spaces in your home always wakeful, and the sleeping places in your home always for sleeping. In other words, only sleep in your bed!

OPTIMIZING YOUR SLEEP

I did a Facebook live the other day, and the night before, I'd enjoyed a particularly great night of sleep. And folks sure noticed! No fewer than twenty people watching commented on how refreshed and bright I looked. (Gee, I wonder what I look like the rest of the time?!) When someone points out that you look rested, it has an impact, and it reminds us how much better we look and feel when we get enough sleep. The truth is, we easily forget or overlook the importance of sleep, until we aren't getting enough of it. The goal is to work toward getting seven-plus hours of sleep a night, as consistently as possible.

In addition to the tips I shared at the top of this chapter, here are some strategies for optimal sleep that you can start implementing and testing out in your own routine.

- Make your bedroom as dark as possible by getting blackout curtains and using black electrical tape to cover tiny LED lights on electronics, smoke detectors, and any other light source.

- Control the temperature in your bedroom so that it isn't varying widely. Typically, 68° to 72°F is a good range.

- Choose lightweight, breathable pajamas that aren't too tight or too loose on your body.

- Make sure your mattress and pillow are comfortable for your body, and not too firm or too soft. If you wake up sore in the morning, it might be time to look at a new mattress.

- Adjust your bedtime slowly, not all at once. If you've been going to bed too late in order to get your seven-plus hours, don't suddenly go to bed two hours earlier one night. Change your bedtime in half-hour increments and give yourself time to get used to it.

- Find a relaxing, calming, meditative activity you can do in the half hour before you want to be asleep. It could be reading, doing breathing exercises, gentle stretching, praying, writing in your journal, or anything else that helps your mind go into a calm state.

- Diffuse lavender essential oil in your bedroom, or use a lavender spray. Lavender has been shown to help promote relaxation.

- If you find yourself lying in your bed unable to sleep, and you've been awake for fifteen minutes or longer, get up and go to a wakeful room, such as the living room. Read a book, play cards, knit, do any kind of activity that requires your attention and not a screen. After fifteen or twenty minutes, if you're feeling sleepy, try going back to bed.

- Avoid daytime napping unless it is in your bed—and if you're having trouble sleeping at night, definitely cut out daytime naps.

Now that you've gotten some ideas for how to improve your sleep habits, it's time to put them into practice. It starts by writing down your game plan.

What possible changes can you make to your nighttime routine or sleeping environment to set yourself up for a better night's sleep?

_____

_____

_____

_____

Once you've tried these tactics for two or three nights, return to the questionnaire on page 109 and see how things have changed. Acknowledge your progress along the way. And keep in mind that your sleep will naturally improve as you continue to adjust your diet, exercise, and manage your stress appropriately.

Now that you're feeling well-rested, I want to talk about a topic that is often overlooked when it comes to weight loss, and that is your support system. I get so fired up about this concept because it is often the missing piece of the puzzle for those who struggle with forming healthy habits. That's why together, we're going to build the ultimate bench so you can score lots more wins for your health.

BUILDING YOUR BENCH

I believe weight loss is a team sport. It is quicker and more easily accomplished if we have a strong team around us. That's why I want you to spend some time building your bench, so that you'll always have the right people to help you get over that goal line. Those bench players are the ones who can make that critical play, and help you win when you can't do it alone. They can encourage you when you feel discouraged; they can shoulder some responsibility when your plate is too full; they can keep you accountable, inspire you, and put things into perspective. These are just some of the ways your bench can help you win more than you lose. Let's think about how you can create your own dream team to help you get where you want to go.

THE POTHOLES OF LIFE

A couple of years back, I was driving from San Diego up to Los Angeles to see a friend, when suddenly—*bang*—I hit a pothole at 70 mph and blew a tire. I slowly maneuvered across the lanes to the shoulder, got to a relatively safe spot, stopped, and took a breath. Once AAA was on their way, I sat there with cars whizzing by outside, trying to figure out my next move.

Then my phone rang. It was a buddy from a group of friends I'll refer to as the "wine nerds." We love all things wine, and we get together a couple times a month to taste and enjoy wine. While I do consider this buddy a friend, he wouldn't necessarily have been the first person I'd think to call when I'm in trouble. But in this case, he actually called me, so I told him what was going on. Ten minutes later, he was there to pick me up from the side of the road. We ended up going to lunch and having a great day. He really got me out of a bind and turned what seemed like a crappy turn of events into an unexpectedly positive one.

We don't always know what role someone will play on our bench until they're needed. The potholes of life give us a chance to be a little vulnerable and ask for help. I know asking for help can be hard, or even embarrassing at times. But think about a time in your life when you've been there for someone and helped them. How awesome did that feel? Now think about how you could give someone else that feeling by allowing them to help you when you need it. The truth is, we often get more out of *giving* assistance than receiving it. So never hesitate to ask for help.

Our game plan has to change and evolve sometimes. You might wake up thinking it's going to be a great day, but then the babysitter calls in sick, or your partner at work gets fired, or any manner of unexpected mayhem occurs, and suddenly your great day goes right down the toilet. This is when you call upon key players on your bench to help you turn things around and get back on track.

And sometimes it's not so much a pothole as a giant sinkhole that suddenly appears and threatens to swallow us whole. My divorce is a perfect example. And for that, I called in my first string, the star player on my team of life, and that's my best friend, Cody. We've known each other since we were in the first grade, and we still talk every week. So it's no surprise that he knew exactly what to say in order to help me as I grieved the loss of my marriage so I could eventually crawl out of that hole and get my feet back on solid ground.

We all need a Cody—that person or those people who know us well and can act as our lifeline, as our way back to ourselves. Even when I first learned of the diagnosis of necrosis in my hips, it was Cody who helped me wrap my head around how I was going to cope. Certainly, I also called upon the medical professionals on my team, and they advised me on the physiological aspects of this newest obstacle in my life. But it was Cody who got me over that emotional piece of the puzzle.

Another important player on my own team is Santiago. I refer to him as my Yoda. We met completely randomly about twenty years ago, and have remained close ever since. Santiago is an old, noble soul. He's seventy-seven years old now, and he came to America from Mexico when he was only ten. His uncle brought him to Indiana to work in the fields. It's tough to imagine, but even at that young age, Santiago viewed this as an opportunity of a lifetime. And boy, did he ever seize that opportunity. A consummate overachiever, Santiago sought out an education any way he could, and ultimately, he attended college at the University of California, Berkeley. His list of professional accolades is a mile long, he reads voraciously, and, as a result, he has an incredible philosopher mindset. When I'm facing any kind of dilemma, it's always Santiago who helps me consider it from new angles.

Santiago is someone who has walked in the shoes of adversity and blazed new paths for himself. So when I come to him with any kind of challenge in my own life, he can empathize, and then help me strategize. I am also able to learn from his life story, and to be inspired by what he has achieved. His wisdom is astounding, and I'm truly grateful to have someone like him in my life and on my team. My wish is that everyone could have access to a Santiago. If you do, be sure to treasure that person, and lean on their knowledge and experience.

The bottom line is this: I don't want you to be caught unprepared for unexpected challenges that can throw you off-balance and keep you from the life you truly deserve. Having a solid bench that you can rely on can keep that from happening.

WHO'S ON YOUR TEAM?

Do you have supporters around you who can help you stay focused on what you need to do in order to achieve your goal? Or do you feel a bit like a lone wolf, out there all on your own? The analogy I always like to use with my patients is making your bed. Think about making your bed by yourself, versus making it with someone else helping you. It's an infinitely easier chore when you have help, right? That's what we want to do—make things a bit easier for you, and a bit more automatic. Your team can do that for you.

Let's do a little exercise to find out who you have in your life who could be helpful to you on this journey. Below are some questions to get you thinking about the types of people you might need to call upon. One person might fill several of these roles, or you might have a handful of people for each one. Write down who comes to mind for each of these roles.

Who is someone in your life who could . . .

- Exercise with you on a regular basis: _____
- Help you with meal planning: _____
- Go grocery shopping with you or for you: _____
- Keep you accountable by checking in with you on a regular basis: _____
- Talk you off the ledge when you feel like giving up: _____
- Encourage you when you're feeling overwhelmed: _____
- Be by your side when something unexpected happens in your life: _____
- Listen when you need to vent, without passing any judgment: _____
- Act as your cheerleader, and congratulate you when you hit milestones: _____

- Follow this plan alongside you in solidarity:

  _____

- Pinch-hit with errands or other responsibilities when you're pulled in too many directions: _____

- Babysit or pet-sit when you need it:

  _____

This isn't an exhaustive list, but it should get you thinking about the specific positions you might want to fill on your own bench. Knowing who you can call on when you need help is the first step in creating the kind of support system that can help you crush your goals and keep crushing them for years to come.

BUILDING YOUR VIRTUAL BENCH

In thinking about this ultimate team you're building, don't forget that not every role has to be filled by someone who lives nearby, or even by people that you know personally. The world has changed and we are having more virtual interactions with one another than ever before. There are pros and cons to that reality, but when it comes to creating a support team, this can be a huge advantage.

As I mentioned earlier, the 17 Day Challenge has become an incredibly positive and fun place where you can meet many other people who are putting these principles into practice and seeing amazing results. What started out as a small group of people who had enjoyed success on the 17 Day Diet quickly grew to be a global online support system. People now come to that Facebook page to share their success, to swap ideas for recipes, and to lift each other up. When someone in Indiana is struggling at 3 a.m., they can go to the page and post about it, and someone in Israel might write back right away with some words of encouragement. Again and again, I've seen people come to each other's aid, and the success speaks for itself.

In fact, when I recently asked for some feedback on the platform, one of our challengers, Beth, shared:

"The 17 Day Challenge is not only a program that shows you how to eat well for overall well-being, but also a community/support system of like-minded individuals always there to offer advice or encouragement. I have gained so much more than I ever expected from this program, and the weight loss was just the icing on the cake. I am proud to be a small part of such an amazing group of people from around the world."

Another challenger, Barbara, said:

"This past summer, I went through a difficult time and needed a positive and healthy diversion. I had joined the challenge hoping to lose five pounds, and it changed my emotional status. I had no idea this program would turn my life around for the better. With the combination of Dr. Mike's morning LIVE chats, member support, and daily accountability, I have gained knowledge and understanding of how my body operates. My big reveal was getting off the 'autopilot' mindset of life. To me, this is more than a program to improve your physical health. It's a program that will improve your mental and emotional health as well. I feel like I found a 'home' with this 17 Day Challenge Community which is filled with so many loving, supportive, and encouraging members. It's full of positivity where I can excel at my own pace and be accountable for my actions. I call it a 'safe zone.' This program is etched in my mind and I'm in a happier place because of it. Plus, my weight loss has been remarkable. I really don't see this as a 'diet' but a healthy lifestyle which produces amazing results. I've lost more weight than I ever expected to."

I love how this group has evolved over time, and how supportive people are with one another on this platform. They've never met in person, but that bond is real.

Social media is one way you can build out your bench, but there are other virtual experiences that can support you in your weight loss journey too. From virtual personal training sessions to meal tracking to apps that help you time your intermittent fasting if that's something you're doing, there are endless options out there. If you're realizing that you would benefit from having a life coach or a psychologist on your team, there are telemedicine apps that can offer you those services in a virtual form as well.

My point is this: think about the specific and unique bench you need to build in order to increase your odds of success, and then cast a wide net to find the right team members for you, both in-person and virtual.

DEALING WITH SABOTEURS

I can't tell you how many patients over the years have told me stories about how it seemed everyone in their lives was bent on sabotaging their weight loss efforts. They'll tell me how they wouldn't want to be rude and refuse their mom's homemade pie. Or how they don't want to make separate meals for their spouse, who doesn't want to eat "diet food." Or how it seems like their friends are constantly pushing them to indulge in unhealthy options. The list of excuses goes on and on, and I get it. When we're starting something new, it can be hard for people in our lives to accept that we're making different choices than we used to.

First, I think it's important to realize that the majority of the time, these people in your life are not purposely trying to sabotage your weight loss. They aren't conspiring to set you up for failure. After all, these are people who care about you and want you to be around for a long time! But you might need to give them a little guidance in *how* they can best support you. It can be as simple as saying,

"I'm really excited to make some changes in my life, and to start choosing more of what I know is good for my health, and less of what I know is detrimental to it. So if I turn down an offer to eat out at our normal greasy spoon, or if I don't have some of your delicious dessert, please don't take it personally. And if you'd like to know the types of things I am eating and doing now, or if you want to try it out with me, I'm happy to share this book with you."

You can also prepare yourself for someone's remarks about your weight loss journey. Take a look at this list and put the responses into your own words so they'll be ready to go when or if needed.

Saboteur: I'm glad to see you're finally losing weight. Hope you can keep it off!

You: I appreciate that, but what would help me even more is if you just congratulated me on what I've already accomplished and left it at that.

Saboteur: Are you still on that diet? Have you actually lost weight?

You: I appreciate your interest, but rather than ask me about my weight, maybe ask how I'm feeling.

Saboteur: I hope you don't get hurt with all that exercise you're doing.

You: I've spoken to my trainer and I feel confident that my exercises are healthy for my body. I am working on my mobility and flexibility to prevent injury.

Saboteur: You're changing with all this weight loss. You're not the same person you were before.

You: I don't know what you're specifically referring to, but I feel good, and I would love it if you could be supportive of my efforts to improve my health.

Saboteur: You're disappearing! Are you losing weight too fast?

You: I feel energized and excited by the weight loss, and I just ask that you be encouraging in how you talk to me about it.

Saboteur: Come on, it's your birthday. Haven't you earned a piece of cake?

You: I don't look at food as something to earn, and I know all that sugar will make me feel terrible. So I'm going to pass, thank you!

Saboteur:	There's only one doughnut left; it has your name on it!
You:	As you know, I'm making progress toward my health goals, and a doughnut will not help me on that path. Could you please help me stay on track?
Saboteur:	You used to love my baked goods. Now you turn your nose up at them. I'm insulted!
You:	Please do not take it personally. I'm working really hard to eat more of what improves my health and less of what trips me up. Your baking is delicious, but for right now, I'm going to politely decline.
Saboteur:	Are you allowed to eat that? Is it on your diet?
You:	My diet is varied and healthy, and I feel good about my choices. And I certainly don't guilt myself. If I need your help, though, I'll let you know! Thank you for your concern.

It comes down to drawing some boundaries for your friends and family and helping them understand how they can be a great teammate for you as you create this new lifestyle.

Also remember that you are ultimately responsible for your own choices about your health. So, as you think about the people in your life, realize that they do not hold the power to make you choose what you put into your body. That responsibility rests squarely on your own shoulders. Don't let any excuses stand in the way of your own success.

BEING A GOOD TEAMMATE

I'm a firm believer that you get back what you put out into the world, so if you want to build a supportive, reliable team, then it's imperative that you find ways to be a good teammate for others as well. I think that's the core reason why this Facebook community we've formed does so well in each and every challenge we run. Everyone understands that they get out of it what they put into it, and the more they support others, the more supported they feel.

Since I come from a big family and have so many siblings, I've seen this principle at work in my life since I was a child. We rally around one another, and we work together when facing adversity. I know it doesn't work that way in every family, but think about your broader circles of friends and look for ways you can help them accomplish their own goals. I promise it will draw you closer together and you'll benefit from it just as much as they will.

And speaking of friendship, did you know that being socially active with your friends can have a significant impact on your overall health? In fact, the differences in health between those who regularly engage with friends versus those who tend to be socially isolated are just as notable as those between nonsmokers and smokers, or nonobese and obese people.[1] That's right, friendships are an important key to good health. So finding ways to spend time with your friends, and to be there for them, can help you improve your physical health as well as your mental well-being.

YOUR STORY, YOUR HEALTH

In the 1990s, my friend and colleague Vincent Felitti led a team of researchers in a landmark study called the CDC-Kaiser Adverse Childhood Experiences (ACE) study. They looked at various types of childhood trauma or household dysfunction that occurred in a group of about 13,500 adults and compared that to the participants' health status, disease, and risk behavior. What they discovered was a "strong graded relationship between the breadth of exposure to abuse or household dysfunction during childhood and multiple risk factors for several of the leading causes of death in adults."[2] In other words, when emotional, physical, or sexual abuse occurred in someone's childhood, they were more likely to experience physical health challenges in adulthood.

Further research indicates that exposure to childhood trauma is a dose-dependent risk factor for a wide range of learning, behavioral, and health problems, both during childhood and into adulthood. It's been shown that patients with a history of ACEs are more likely to engage in unhealthy behaviors such as overeating, physical inactivity, and smoking. These patients have been shown to disproportionately experience alcoholism, substance abuse, and depression. People with a history of childhood trauma are also more likely to suffer from sleep disturbances, obesity, diabetes, ischemic heart disease, chronic obstructive airway disease, and cancer as adults. As a result, these patients are also at increased risk of early mortality.[3]

All of this may come as a surprise to you, or it may not, but what I want you to take away from this groundbreaking study, which doctors are still using with patients across the country, is this: your life story very often informs your health. The choices we make regarding our health can stem from experiences we had in childhood. Does that mean we have no control over them? No, of course not. But bringing awareness to connections between behavior and experiences in our lives can be incredibly valuable.

For example, maybe you have been using food as a source of comfort since a young age. Or maybe you tend to choose drugs or alcohol as coping mechanisms because you don't have healthy tools for dealing with emotional experiences from your past. It could even be that you've been dealing with undiagnosed depression for many years, and that in and of itself has had an adverse effect on your health.

First, I hope that you will forgive yourself for unhealthy behaviors and never beat yourself up for them. Adding guilt to the equation is simply counterproductive. Second, if there is something that you haven't fully faced or dealt with from your adolescence, I hope you will seek help. There are so many resources available; all it takes is for you to reach out and bring someone onto your team who has the skills to help you heal those wounds. You didn't have any control over what happened to you as a child, but now you are writing your own life story. So ask yourself: What will be in the next chapter? If the book I've been writing up until now isn't going the way I want it to, what can I do to change the story now?

YOUR FOURTH QUARTER

Whether you're a sports player or a fan, you likely know the saying: *The game is won or lost in the fourth quarter*. The same is true when our goal is weight loss and restoring our health. It's not about what we accomplish in the first few days; it's about what we do in the long run. I want you to be able to permanently put away that yo-yo diet mentality, because what good does it really do you in the span of your life to just keep losing the same ten or twenty pounds over and over? I want you to be able to unlock a new reality that allows you to enjoy your life and not have to focus obsessively on what you're eating or how much you're exercising. I want to help you automate those things you need to do in order to improve and maintain your weight and health. A big part of how we accomplish that is to hone your team around you.

Take a moment now and look back at your list of teammates that you started earlier in this chapter, and determine whether you need to add any roles or people to that list. While reading this chapter, has someone come to mind whom you could be leaning on for a specific type of support? Write it down so that you can come here anytime and be reminded of just how strong your bench truly is. Let this be something you continue to work on so that your team can continue to evolve as your life does.

In the next chapter, I'm going to share with you the most practical, useful strategies for dealing with the number-one biggest obstacle to both weight loss and good health: stress. These are stressful times, for sure, but I have seen these methods work time and again, and I am convinced they'll work for you too.

WINNING YOUR BATTLE WITH STRESS

Resilience is more important when it comes to stress than in any other area of life. Why? Because stress is inevitable. You can't run and you can't hide; stress will find a way in. To try to "avoid" stress is unreasonable. And I don't know about you, but anytime someone tells me, "Don't let stress get to you," it just makes me stress out even more. The key is to build up resiliency so that when stress does hit, you're able to manage it and still maintain your health—because make no mistake, stress can have a significant impact on your health if you allow it.

There's an old saying that stress will kill you, and unfortunately, it is actually accurate. It can be a slow, painful way to go down too. Stress can become chronic and debilitating. Just to give you a better idea of its effects on your physiology, here are the highlights:

- Chronic stress is when your body's natural "fight or flight" stress response never really shuts off, and your body is constantly releasing hormones such as adrenaline and cortisol, which can be harmful when released over long periods of time.

- Remaining in that state for an extended period, rather than only briefly as nature intended, means your body is constantly being exposed to elevated levels of these hormones, which affects every single bodily function.

- According to the Mayo Clinic, this hormonal cascade can lead to:
  - Anxiety
  - Depression
  - Digestive problems
  - Headaches
  - Heart disease
  - Sleep problems
  - Weight gain
  - Memory and concentration impairment[1]

Need I go on? Stress is insidious, there's no question about it. And I see it every day in my office. When my patients come in complaining of anything from chronic headaches to gastrointestinal issues, from lethargy or trouble sleeping to recent weight gain or joint pain, or just about anything else, once we get to talking we often realize that stress is at the root. Maybe you've noticed that pattern in your own health too.

One afternoon I was seeing a patient named Will, and as we went through his list of symptoms, I asked if he had been dealing with any new stresses. With a big sigh and a frown that seemed to take over his entire face, he started unloading. He told me that about six months prior, he'd run into some financial problems, and ever since then he was constantly worrying about something. He said it wasn't always money that was troubling him; his mind was just always occupied with stressful thoughts. It was clear that he didn't have a method for coping with all of it, so I gave him an example I've given countless other patients. I said, "Okay, I have a hypothetical question. What if you let the weather patterns determine how your day was going to go? How would that work?"

He said, "Well, that would be crazy."

And I said, "Right. Now, let's say you watch the weather report, and the forecast calls for rain and cold temperatures tomorrow. You can't change that it's going to be rainy and cold. The weather is going to do what it's going to do. But you can take an umbrella or wear a jacket. My point is this: don't ignore what's going on completely because that doesn't help, but don't stress about it either. Get the information and then do what you can do, what you have *control* over. Then you'll know you've done what you could and you no longer need to stress about it." As I was talking, he began to visibly relax his body.

"I think that's been my problem," he said. "I've just been stuck in my head about everything. I haven't been able to get out from under it. I've been trying to change the weather, I guess you could say. But doing what I can about it and then moving on is better. It will be a relief actually."

"Good," I said, "give it a try and then report back."

When I saw Will a month later, his wife was with him in the exam room when I walked in. The second I opened the door, she stood up, came over to me, and shook my hand. I was a little caught off guard, and before I could say anything, she blurted out, "Thank you so much, Doctor, for giving me back my husband."

I laughed, looked over at him, and said, "So, it seems our plan is working."

He sheepishly smiled and replied, "Apparently my stress was affecting everyone in the household." His wife nodded intensely.

"It has a way of doing that. But I'm happy for both of you. Keep up the good work." I was so pleased to see that he'd been better managing everything that was stressing him out, as indicated both by his test results (which showed a reduction in his blood pressure, and a full ten pounds of weight loss in just four weeks), and by his wife's show of appreciation.

You see, one of the aspects of stress that we often overlook is that it's contagious. Just like any virus or other pathogen we encounter, stress can be passed to others around us. When we're really feeling the pressure, we don't have as much patience, so we snap at our family members. We aren't ourselves. We're overly tired, grumpy, and disengaged. If we let it go on too long, then we begin to look at everything through a lens of negativity. And it's really hard for people in our lives to stay optimistic when they're around us in that state. So relationships start to degrade. And as the downward spiral continues, those we're living with begin to experience many of the same symptoms of chronic stress that we do. Brutal.

There is good news, though. Stress might be a fact of our modern life, but that doesn't mean it has to *rule* your life. Starting right now, you can begin to build up your resilience so that you don't experience its detrimental health effects. You can take the power back into your own hands so that you aren't a prisoner to stress. And since chronic stress, in my opinion, is one of the top reasons why people can't lose weight and keep it off, it's imperative that you make this a priority in your life if you're looking to drop some pounds and inches.

YOUR STRESS BATTLE STRATEGY

Very often, when we're feeling the mental effects of stress, it's because we are worrying about things that are beyond our control. We spend lots of time and brainpower on them, yet there's absolutely nothing we can do to change them. As a result, they stay in our consciousness and fester. Like an infected cut, they just get worse and make us sicker. You need a clear-cut strategy for preventing this.

The first step is to acknowledge the things that are causing you to stress. There's a mental satiety or comfort that comes from saying out loud, "This is a stress in my life." By naming it, you are acknowledging its existence instead of just letting it linger in the back of your mind, or allowing it to ride on your mental merry-go-round of negative thoughts. Merely giving it five or ten seconds of acknowledgment can go a long way.

The next step is to create a stress inventory. You write down everything that is stressing you out, but you divide the list into two categories: avoidable stress and unavoidable stress.

WHAT IS UNAVOIDABLE STRESS?

Referring back to the story I told you about my patient Will, you can think about unavoidable stressors as being like the weather. You have zero control over what the weather will do, but you can prepare and plan for it. Examples include things that haven't happened yet, and maybe they never will, but that you are worried about. Maybe you're concerned about your child or another family member getting hurt, or maybe you worry about your own health. Perhaps you're afraid of losing your job in uncertain times, or about your finances in general.

Next to each item on your unavoidable stress list, write down what you can do to help mitigate this stress. If you're worried about your job, consider updating your résumé one evening, or doing some networking so that you have a backup plan in place. If you fret about some particular aspect of your health, you can do some research to find out how you can prevent a certain illness or issues. If it's a family member you worry about a lot, maybe there's a discussion you can have with those who care for them when you aren't around.

Finally, if you've done all you can to prepare for or prevent a particular stress, you can use breathing exercises or other coping skills that I'll outline below. At a certain point, we all have to learn to let go and stop trying to control so much in our lives, and I will help you do that.

WHAT IS AVOIDABLE STRESS?

The avoidable stress list includes the types of worries that you can actually do something about. There is some kind of action that you can take on these items that will make them feel less stressful, or remove them from your list entirely. Some examples include work assignments, family get-togethers, unaddressed health issues, and so on. You can take steps toward completing these things hanging over your head—and when you do, you start to feel less stressed out about them. If there's an assignment you've been putting off, and the longer you do the worse it feels, just carve out some time and get it done. Or if you have an event coming up that you haven't planned for at all, make your to-do list and start knocking it out. That's how you make these stressors into "avoidable stress"—by taking action.

Next to your avoidable stress items, you will write down what you can do to avoid feeling stressed out about each one—creating time in your schedule to finish a project, asking for help, **making a doctor's appointment, doing prep work, and so on. When you take action toward** completing a task that feels like it's looming overhead, **you automatically feel less stressed. It's all about *action*.**

Now it's your turn to give it a try. Write down your **current stressors and** what you can do to manage them in the following **chart.**

My Stress Inventory

Avoidable Stress	Ways I Can Avoid It

Unavoidable Stress	Ways I Can Prepare for, Prevent, or Cope with It

Return to this exercise daily if you need to. I know people who fill out a chart like this every morning while drinking their coffee. For others, it's a tool they only use when they're feeling especially overwhelmed. It's up to you, but this is an extremely valuable tool for winning your own battle with stress.

LETTING IT GO

So, you've done everything you possibly can to prevent or prepare for an unavoidable stress, and you still can't stop thinking about it. We've all been there. This is when we have to lean on tried-and-true coping mechanisms that help us let go of worry. For me, exercise is key. I believe exercise is the best prescription for stress. Anything you can do to get your heart rate up is going to help you take your mind off your worries. Walking, jogging, dancing, jumping jacks or other plyometric exercises, lifting weights or any form of resistance training—it's all good for stress management, especially when done on a regular basis.

As I've shared with you, I'm an avid swimmer. It is my favorite form of destressing. A big part of why I think swimming gives me such stress relief has to do with the rhythmic breathing it requires. But you don't have to plunge into the pool to enjoy the benefits of purposeful breath work. You can do it in your car, in the shower, while preparing a meal, lying in bed, even sitting at your desk. It's very simple, and highly effective. Try it right now by following this breathing pattern, which is called "box breathing":

De-Stress with Breath

1. If you are seated, make sure you aren't hunched over. Keep your shoulders back and your chest up.

2. Inhale slowly through your nose for a count of four seconds. While breathing in, expand your stomach out so that you are activating your diaphragm. Keep your shoulders as still as you can during the breath.

3. Hold for a count of four. If that's too long, hold for two or three seconds, and work your way up to four.

4. Exhale through your nose for a count of four, while pulling your stomach in toward your belly button.

5. Rest for a count of four.

6. Repeat until you feel your mind quieting and your heart rate normalizing.

That's a go-to anytime you need to relax your nervous system and get out of a state of fight-or-flight. But I will say, it requires practice. Though it might appear to be a simple exercise when you read it on paper, it's not always that easy when you try it. You might find yourself yawning a lot at first. Trust me, it gets better the more you practice it. Try to fit it in several times a day, and you'll be surprised how much easier it becomes over time.

By the way, you can use this technique during a workout. If you find yourself huffing and puffing, or feeling like your lungs are going to explode when you're trying a new form of cardio, stop and do your four-counts of breath. It will quickly bring you back to normal breathing, and then you can jump back into your workout.

Another great method to try out is a visualization technique. Here's how it goes:

Visualize Your Calm
1. Imagine you are standing barefoot on soft grass.

2. Then think about a warm, healing light hovering above your head.

3. The light moves down over and around your head, then slowly through your body.

4. Take several seconds to think about, focus on, and deeply relax each part of your body as the light slowly moves through your head and brain, your face and sinuses, then your neck, shoulders, arms, hands and fingers, chest, lungs and heart, abdomen, digestive system, pelvis, reproductive system and urinary tract, hips, upper legs, knees, lower legs, ankles, and feet and toes.

5. The more you can envision this warm, healing light touching every part of your body, the more awareness and calmness you bring to each of your body systems.

This is an effective tool in helping yourself detach from stress and bring a sense of peace and calm to your entire body. There are lots of different variations on guided visualizations that you can find online or in apps for your phone. I highly recommend giving this technique a try, because it harnesses the power of your mind and can help you gain mastery over stress.

Meditation is another great stress reliever; like these other techniques, it's something you can do every day to really unlock its maximum benefits. When I was growing up, I was an altar boy in church. And I was always that kid who prayed with one eye open. I just couldn't make myself go inward and pray silently; I had to know what was going on around me. This tendency carried through into my adult life, and as a result, I've always struggled with meditation. So if it's tough for you, too, know that you're not alone.

I know a lot of people think meditation is hard, and that's because all day long, we are so used to sensory overload. We have information coming in from multiple sources, and our minds are always flying from one thought to another. Meditation means seeking silence within the mind. And it requires practice. But even if you're never able to fully quiet your mind, taking time to just sit in silence is still great for releasing some stress. Here are some tips for meditating:

Meditation 101

1. Plan to meditate for one minute if you're a first-timer. You can aim to work up to thirty minutes or more per day, but it's always wise to start with shorter periods of time.

2. Find as quiet and comfortable a place to sit as you can.

3. Place your feet flat on the floor if you're on a chair or sit cross-legged on the ground.

4. Begin to breathe slowly, and gently close your eyes.

5. Choose a word or sound that has no specific meaning to you, or even make up a new word. Some people like to use "om" or "mmm." Let that sound or word be your primary thought for this one-minute session.

6. Inevitably, thoughts will begin to enter your mind. So imagine that each thought is a leaf. Place the leaf on a gently flowing river and let it float away in the water.

7. Continue breathing slowly and releasing thought leaves into the river until the time is up.

8. Realize that there is no right or wrong way to meditate. Even if you weren't able to slow the flow of thoughts, it was still a successful meditation. Over time, you will be able to find more and more quiet in your mind.

It's all about starting where you are and progressing forward as you feel comfortable. Simply by sitting down, turning off distractions, and being in silence, you are already resetting your sympathetic and parasympathetic nervous systems. You're getting that fight-or-flight impulse back into balance. So even if you don't feel like you are truly "meditating," don't worry. Meditation is hard because it's supposed to be hard. Running a marathon is hard, but walking a block is not. You run a marathon by first walking blocks. With anything in life, there's training involved, and meditation is no different.

And remember, learning to let go of stress requires a daily commitment. The more you choose to let it go by using whatever technique works for you, the easier it will become.

Wendy's Stress Story

Wendy Epps is one of the community members on the 17 Day Challenge I have going on Facebook. When I asked the community for feedback on the program, she wrote something I just had to share with you. Wendy said, "This lifestyle has changed the way I look at food, it has given me the mindset to no longer use food as a stress relief and enjoy it instead. I now use exercise and meditation as my stress relief and it's paying off with a healthy mind and body." Right on, Wendy! Keep up the great work.

BOTTLING JOY

Wouldn't it be nice to have an immediate antidote anytime stress starts to make you feel funky? Like a little bottle of joy that you could just drink from whenever you need it, but without any side effects? Well, I recently discovered exactly how to do that, and I am excited to share it with you.

I was on a cruise vacation not long ago, and we were hanging out and relaxing in the bar area before dinner. The bartender, who was a true performer, did a trick while making a martini that was so funny and unexpected; it just struck me as hilarious. I was cracking up at that and feeling the complete, utter joy you experience when you're hitting pause on work for a few days and taking in the slack. I didn't realize it, but my girlfriend snapped a picture of me in that exact moment.

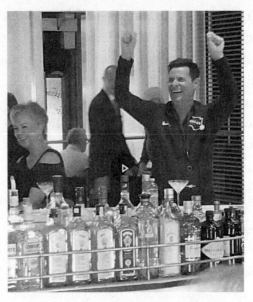

Did I just witness the winning touchdown of the Super Bowl, or watch a bartender make a martini? You decide!

A couple weeks after the vacation was over, I was having dinner after a nonstop day at work and I received a text message from my girlfriend. It was that photo. I couldn't believe it. The second I looked at it, I recalled that feeling and felt pure joy coursing through my veins. It was as if I was right back there on the cruise. And I had an epiphany. Anytime I wanted to, I could revisit that and other happy memories in my mind and enjoy the same chemical release of endorphins in my brain as when I actually lived them. I realized: it is completely possible to bottle joy and drink from it again and again.

Conduct your own joy experiment right now by closing your eyes and imagining a moment in your own life when you felt truly, deeply happy. Maybe it was at a birthday party when you were ten years old, surrounded by friends and family as you blew out the candles on your cake. Or perhaps it was lying on a beach listening to the waves gently lap at the shore. The first time you ever held your child or grandchild in your arms. Or dancing the night away with good friends. Paint the whole picture in your mind, and think about every detail you can recall. Breathe in and out deeply as you revisit that moment in time.

In fact, write a few of these moments down. It's always so easy to write a list of the things that are stressing us out, but it takes a little more digging to recall the moments that gave us pure bliss. Or it could be a favorite movie or book. Whenever I've had a tough day, I always put on the movie *Sideways*. It makes me laugh and brings me back to calm.

Take the time right now to write down what's in your bottle of joy so that you can have quick access to it whenever you need it.

My Bottle of Joy

1. _____
2. _____
3. _____
4. _____
5. _____
6. _____
7. _____
8. _____
9. _____
10. _____

Now, after having thought about those moments, how do you feel? Happier? More relaxed? Remember, these memories do not simply exist in the past. You can recall them anytime you wish and access the rejuvenating and invigorating feelings they produce. When the stress and pressure of the day are getting to you, or you need to break out of a negative thought pattern, simply have a sip from your very own bottle of joy.

I often play a game called "Remember When" with my lifelong buddy Cody, whom I told you about earlier. All of a sudden, in the middle of the week or even the middle of the night, he'll text me and say, "Remember when . . ." and then recall one of the countless funny memories from our past. Anytime I open a text and see those words, I get so excited. I know I'm in for a good laugh.

Recently, I got one of those texts and it said, "Remember when...I'll give you a dollar if you can throw me out of your room." Instantly, I went back in time to when we were just fourteen years old, freshmen in high school. Every weekend we traded off staying at each other's houses, and I was so annoyed that he always wanted to go to bed by 11 p.m. I mean, what freshman kid goes to bed that early on a Saturday night? I wanted to at least stay up long enough to finish watching *Saturday Night Live*. But not Cody. He would get up from the living room couch just before 11 p.m. every weekend, and head straight to bed. Well, one night, I simply wasn't going to allow it.

After he'd gotten settled into his twin bed, and I was supposed to be getting into the other one, I walked over to him and said, "I'll give you a dollar if you can throw me out of your room." He barely peeked through one eye at me, and promptly turned over, pulling the covers up over his head. Now, mind you, Cody was bigger than me, by a lot. But I didn't care. I was bored and unrelenting.

"Come on, man! I'll give you a dollar," I said as I started poking at him and loudly stomping around. Finally he'd had enough. Cody leaped out of bed, grabbed me by the shirt, chucked me into the hallway, and locked the door behind me. I was laughing the whole time, loving how riled up he got. So, of course, once he let me back in a couple minutes later, I did it again, only this time, I was stacking feathers from my pillow on his forehead, poking him with the feathers, challenging him, daring him, and, yes, promising him another dollar if he could do it again.

By the time he'd successfully thrown me out of his room three times in a row (and I'd dragged the sheets on his bed with me that third time), his mom finally came to see what the ruckus was all about. And I, with all the skill and knowledge of a seasoned little brother, managed to get Cody in trouble for "locking me out of his room and not letting me back in." Ha! My mischief paid off, and I got to stay up late.

Reliving silly moments like that is like tonic for the soul. It's my favorite kind of stress reliever. Do you have any great "remember when" stories you could remind someone of? You might just make their day... and your own.

STRESSPROOFING YOUR LIFE

We are busier these days than ever before, and all that running around and knocking items off the to-do list can really take a toll if you're not careful. But you don't have to let it all get to you. A little planning goes a long way.

Here are some stress hacks to try out:

- **Protect Your Sleep Routine:** Your body needs adequate rest each day, and that's especially true when you're putting the pedal to the metal with work, family, even holiday times. Set regular bedtimes and stick with them no matter what. In fact, you can even set your phone alarm to go off at a certain time each night so you're reminded to start your ready-for-bed routine. This should include some quiet time to wind down from the day, maybe have a cup of chamomile tea, and anything else that helps you relax for a great night's sleep. The best defender against the ravaging effects of stress is good, regular sleep.

- **Keep It Reasonable:** When your stress levels are through the roof because of extraordinary circumstances (such as a loss, a family member's health challenges, a big move, losing a job, etc.), avoid putting added pressure on yourself to lose weight during these times. Instead, set some realistic goals about continuing to incorporate more of what you know is good for your health (i.e., time spent moving your body) and less of what is harmful to it (I'm looking at you, cheesecake). You can focus on weight loss again once the dust has settled a bit in your life.

- **Boost Your M&M Practice:** It's easy to lose sight of your motivations and your mindfulness when you're feeling the stress squeeze. But ironically, this is the time when you most need that M&M to help you stay healthy and feeling good. So try to be intentional about connecting with your motivations first thing each morning.

The moment you open your eyes, remind yourself why you're focusing on your health more than ever. Those deep motivations will help inspire you along the way and keep you from getting lost in the stress fray. Also, try to be present in each moment rather than constantly rushing on to the next thing, and the next. Take slow, relaxing breaths, and tune into what you are grateful for in life.

- **Send Guilt Packing:** If there's one unwelcome guest in your life, it's guilt. Even if you get yourself a bit off track, maybe overindulging in dessert or having a little too much to drink, don't let guilt make matters worse. Instead, make a health decision right away. That might mean going for a walk, doing some yoga, having a cup of green tea, or meditating for five minutes. Choosing to make the next right step in the direction of your health will be so much more productive than wallowing in guilt.

- **Prioritize and Delegate:** Instead of trying to do it all and be everything for everyone, prioritize what's really important to you and tackle those things first. And then, delegate! I received the best advice from a friend once, and that was to "only do the things that only you can do." If there's someone in your family who could help you with some aspect of what needs to get done, by all means, delegate that task! There are all kinds of apps these days that allow you to pay a nominal fee for someone to do your shopping, stand in line, and do other personal tasks. It's definitely worth looking into.

- **When in Doubt, Hydrate:** Drink. More. Water. Have a bottle of water with you at all times. I'm not kidding! Especially if you live in a cold climate, staying hydrated is vitally important. Keeping your body hydrated can also reduce the effects of stress, prevent headaches, and help you flush out any toxins from foods. And if you do have a cocktail or two, be sure to drink one glass of water for every 1 ounce of liquor, 6 ounces of wine, or 8 ounces of beer that you consume. Trust me, you'll thank me in the morning.

SAVING UP

As you continue onward toward your health and weight goals, you can begin to think of your health as a savings account. You are always making deposits into it or withdrawals from it. When you give in to stress and let it take over your mind and body, you are withdrawing some big-time health bucks. If you're not careful, you can go bankrupt really quickly.

On the other hand, when you are committed to winning your battles with stress, you are making deposits into your health account. You're protecting your body from the damage stress can cause, and boosting your bottom line. The more health "dollars" you have saved up, the better you will feel overall.

In the next chapter, we're going to talk about another great way to increase your health savings so that you can lose weight more easily, experience less inflammation, and much, much more. I can't wait to dive into this topic with you.

THE CBD REVOLUTION

When I first had the idea to write this book, it was because of the information I am going to be revealing in this chapter. I had just discovered the amazing power of CBD (short for cannabidiol) and I was on fire. I still am! The emerging research is promising, and the success stories I've heard from many of the people who tried out CBD supplements and muscle rubs during my 17 Day Challenge are nothing short of astounding. From pain relief to a reduction in symptoms of anxiety, from improved sleep to less inflammation, the list of ways CBD can improve our quality of life just goes on and on. And I know this because I've experienced it firsthand.

When I first started dealing with chronic pain and I was working with my physicians to discover the source, I was taking maximum doses of over-the-counter pain meds and a prescription medication for inflammation. I didn't like being on all those meds, and my body didn't either. They would work for a while, but inevitably I'd end up on the floor of my office, trying desperately to relieve the pressure on my back. The pain was disrupting my sleep, and it was tough to be the best version of myself at work. I needed a real solution without intense side effects . . . fast.

And then I was reminded of CBD, which I had been intrigued by years before but had never really tried for myself. As you've probably noticed by now, I'm not someone who just jumps onto bandwagons without doing my homework. So I dove headlong into the available research, and sought the advice of experts. I knew some people were skeptical because CBD is derived from the marijuana plant. There's somewhat of a stigma because it comes from "pot." But given that I believe so strongly in a plant-forward diet, and that I'm very familiar with the medicinal power certain plants can hold, I was not one of those skeptics. In fact, I have a bit of a "get over it" mentality when it comes to that particular objection to CBD. I believe the best medication in the world is no medication, and the second-best is one from a natural source that helps you, doesn't harm you, and doesn't break the bank. For those reasons, CBD was right up my alley.

The more I read about it and talked to folks who had used it or other doctors who had seen success with it, the more convinced I became. I tried it. And right away, within the first few days, I could tell it was already helping with my sleep. And then, after using it for about a month, I started to notice it was having a positive impact on my mood and my pain. I've discovered that the length of time it takes for CBD to work differs for everyone; some people notice a difference right away, while for others the effects kick in later. But I encourage people to try it for at least six weeks before determining whether it will work for them or not. For me, it was at the five-week mark that I knew without a doubt CBD was going to be a game changer. And it was well worth the wait. Once I was more rested and feeling less overall pain, I started to work in some regular acupuncture and chiropractic treatments from trusted practitioners, and the combination got me to a place where my pain is very manageable, and some days now I have none at all.

The biggest conundrum with CBD is that we can't know for sure whether it will work on someone before they try it. Some of us are just not sensitive to exogenous forms. Not everything is explicable in medicine, unfortunately. But because there are no negative side effects, there's no real risk in trying it for yourself. It's not going to hurt you in any way, whereas prescription pain medications, such as opioids, definitely could.

I've been recommending CBD to many of my patients, and I'd say that in at least 80 percent, it has some positive effect. Look at it this way: if we were talking about buying a stock, and there was zero risk of losing money and a strong possibility of making money, everyone in the world would do it. Think of it as an investment in your health.

If you're curious about how CBD has supported other people on their journey to lose weight and feel better in their lives, check out these rave reviews:

• • • • • • •

"The CBD drops have helped me to fall asleep quickly and sleep through the night. Previously, it would take me a long time to fall asleep and I would frequently wake up during the night. With the drops, I immediately began sleeping better, giving me more energy for my workouts and day-to-day tasks."
—CASSANDRA PAVEL

"I have pain in my legs and feet all the time; the CBD cream has been fantastic. I use it often for better mobility. I am able to exercise more consistently because I have less pain. I am burning more calories which helps on my weight loss journey. I rest really well when using the drops, without the 'drugged' feeling I often get with over-the-counter sleep aids. I will be forever grateful to Dr. Mike for the gift of these products. Dr. Mike's books and these products have definitely impacted my life in very positive ways."
—BETSY BRAUSER ACKLEY

"The CBD definitely helps with my sleep. My issue is staying asleep or falling back to sleep after waking up and nothing else has worked as well for this. I take regular CBD daily during the day and it really helps keep anxiety at bay. It also helps my mood stability so that I'm more apt to make healthy choices."
—TRINA DAVIDSON

• • • • • • •

Pretty compelling, right? Now I'll walk you through the basics so you can gain enough of an understanding to feel comfortable with considering adding it to your supplementation routine.

ENDOCANNABA...WHAT?

In case you're wondering, even though CBD is derived from the marijuana plant, it does not get you "high." THC, short for tetrahydrocannabinol, is the cannabinoid that produces psychoactive effects. So you don't need to worry about experiencing any of those side effects when you use CBD. In order to understand how CBD works in the body, you first have to know a little bit about the endocannabinoid system (ECS). Unlike organ systems (such as your cardiovascular system or digestive system), the ECS is a biochemical communication system. It's made up of receptors that exist in cells throughout the body, from neurons to immune cells. The main function of the ECS is to help your body maintain homeostasis. It kicks into high gear anytime you are injured or sick, to help you get back to your baseline.[1]

The ECS is a very complex system, and researchers don't yet know everything there is to know about it. But we do know that cannabidiol (CBD), as well as more than a hundred other cannabinoids from the marijuana plant, interacts with the body's ECS. And CBD has been shown to have potent effects on the human body, including antitumor, antioxidant, antispasmodic, antipsychotic, anticonvulsive, and neuroprotective properties. CBD also activates serotonin receptors, which results in an antianxiety effect.[2] Bottom line—it can help with a wide range of health issues, both by reducing symptoms and by speeding healing.

OKAY, BUT WHAT DOES CBD
HAVE TO DO WITH LOSING WEIGHT?

A lot! As we've been talking about, weight loss is not simply a matter of food and exercise. There are many other factors that play into our ability to get to a healthy weight and remain there. CBD can help with several of those factors. Of course, I'm not saying that CBD is a silver bullet for losing weight. It isn't a weight loss miracle in a bottle. But it is a supplement that has a lot of promise for improving your chances of losing weight, and without worrisome side effects. Here are some of the ways it can be helpful in your journey:

Catching Your Zzz's

Healthy sleep is critical to healthy weight loss. Period. If you changed nothing else about your lifestyle other than improving your sleep, I'm willing to bet you would lose weight. And according to recent studies, CBD may help you fall asleep and stay asleep.[3]

Reducing Pain so You Can Move

We know that daily movement can help with weight loss and improving your health. But if you're dealing with chronic pain, exercise is probably the last thing you feel like doing. CBD might be able to help. It has been shown to have analgesic effects on various chronic pain conditions.[4] I've been using it to manage pain in my body for over a year now, and I can personally vouch for its effectiveness. Because I have less pain, I'm able to exercise more often and for longer periods. Of course, it doesn't work exactly the same way for everyone, but it's definitely worth trying.

Stabilizing Appetite

Unlike THC, which has been known to produce an effect on your appetite commonly referred to as "the munchies," CBD does not appear to stimulate the appetite. On the contrary, according to animal studies, certain anti-inflammatory properties of CBD may actually help reduce food intake.[5] This is because inflammation in the body can trigger certain hormones that make you feel hungry or crave sugary foods. So when you reduce inflammation, you reduce those cravings, and thus you don't tend to overeat or reach for those unhealthy foods. Studies also show that CBD helps convert white fat cells into brown fat cells, a more active form of fat that actually burns calories.

Regulating Mood

If you tend to overeat, or to reach for comfort food or junk food when you're feeling sad or stressed or in any other heightened emotional state, CBD might be able to help you out there too. It has been shown to have a calming effect on the central nervous system, which can alleviate anxiety.[6] In a study on CBD's effect on anxiety and sleep for seventy-two adults at a psychiatric clinic over three months, 66.7 percent of patients reported better sleep and 79.2 percent reported decreased anxiety. More studies are needed, but I find the initial findings to be promising.

HOW DO I TAKE CBD?

Okay, so you want to know how you can start incorporating CBD into your lifestyle, but you have no idea where to start. Been there! It's not quite as straightforward as some other types of supplements, so it's going to require some trial and error on your part. I'll first let you know it's important to discuss your plans to take CBD with your physician. While CBD does not usually carry with it any contraindications, running it by your doctor is always wise for added peace of mind.

I take two different oral tinctures, which is a liquid form of CBD that comes with a dropper—a morning tincture and a nighttime one. The nighttime tincture also has valerian root, melatonin, and other elements that are sleep-promoting. The morning one is only CBD, and it is around 300 mg. There are different dosages available, so read the package about the dose range. CBD dosage is a bell-shaped curve, and there's a sweet spot in the middle.

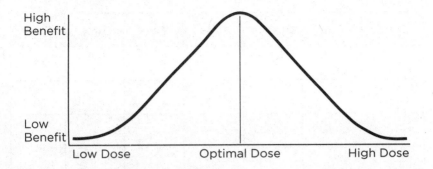

I also use a muscle rub with CBD in it, because it gets absorbed through the skin. I use it on sore areas such as my neck, lower back, and any muscles that are sore after I work out. There are lotions, serums, balms, gels, and other topical applications available. These can really help with localized pain. So, for instance, if you're experiencing low-back pain, you can rub some directly into the painful area. Same goes for joints, etc. I even know someone who uses it on her temples and the base of her skull for headaches. Now, if you're using it all day long, it can definitely get expensive, but what I've found is that it doesn't take much to be effective.

Transdermal patches have become quite popular, too, so you might consider that modality. Typically, absorption is comparable to taking the supplement orally, but because you're wearing the patch all day, the CBD is delivered over a longer period of time, and more evenly.[7]

In order to know whether CBD products are working for me, I've found it helpful to keep a log of which products I'm taking, what dosage, and how often. I use a chart like this one below. I highly recommend you keep track so that you can begin to understand what works best for you. You can track oral/sublingual supplementation, as well as any topical treatments you're using.

Product Name	Dosage	Date	Time	Time	Time

HOW TO CHOOSE YOUR CBD SUPPLEMENTS

Knowing that you're getting on a good product is the most important factor when it comes to choosing which form and brand of CBD you're going to use. As with any supplement out there, you'll find high-quality versions and lower-quality versions. The advice I always give is to check the label and make sure the ingredients have been reviewed by a third-party agency. For example, the USP verified mark certifies that what is on the label is actually in the bottle.[8] The USP (United States Pharmacopeia) is an independent, nonprofit organization that tests medicines and supplements to be sure these items are properly labeled. It's a good idea to purchase products that have been verified—otherwise, there really is no regulation or oversight. And I've heard about a handful of products that advertise CBD as an ingredient, but testing revealed none at all in the actual formulation. Buyer beware!

Full disclosure: I have been a spokesperson for a company called OptaNaturals, and I use their CBD product line. Again, there are lots of options out there, so you should do your homework and even try a few different ones. But I wanted to share with you the particular brand I have gravitated toward, as that has been a question I've received a lot from patients and via social media channels.

I encourage you to consider incorporating CBD supplementation into your lifestyle. I really believe it can be helpful to you as you start to lose weight and restore your overall health. It has certainly done that for me!

GOOOOOOAL(S)!!!

This is usually the part of a diet book where you think about your goal weight—if you're getting close to it, what it will feel like when you reach it, and how you'll then maintain that goal while still living your life. Well, as you likely noticed, this plan is a little different. Our goal is not simply a static number on a scale. Our journey does not end when your weight tells us it's over. Instead, we are working toward creating a sustainable, overall healthy lifestyle that comprises many different daily goals. You are now going to be a nonstop goal-getter, and it's going to feel so good.

Right now, let's take a fresh look at the quizzes you took in chapter 2. I want you to see how you've already been achieving goals by choosing more positive behavior across the board in just seventeen days. Check back to see what your answers were when you started this diet, and then compare them to your answers today.

YOUR "GETTING STARTED"/"KEEPING IT UP" QUIZ

1. How often do you currently eat or drink the following categories per week: soda (diet or regular), fast food, fried food?
   - Never—0 points

- Very rarely, just once in a while—1 point
- Sometimes—2 points
- Often—3 points
- Several times a day—4 points

2. How often do you currently drink alcohol (beer, wine, liquor, alcoholic seltzers)?
   - Never or very rarely—0 points
   - Only a special occasion—1 point
   - One or two times a week—2 points
   - Three or four times a week—3 points
   - Five-plus times per week on average—4 points

3. How often do you currently eat foods high in sugar (desserts such as ice cream or frozen yogurt, baked goods, candy)?
   - Never or very rarely—0 points
   - Only on a special occasion—1 point
   - One or two times a week—2 points
   - Three or four times a week—3 points
   - Five-plus times per week on average—4 points

4. How often are you eating plant-forward meals, where animal protein makes up 10 percent or less of the total meal?
   - Every meal—0 points
   - Fairly often—1 point
   - Once in a while—2 points
   - Rarely—3 points
   - Never—4 points

5. What is your current relationship with stress?
   - I'm a zen master; I know exactly how to cope when stress comes—0 points
   - It depends on the day; sometimes I tackle stress head-on, and sometimes I'm a total mess—1 point

- I worry about the stuff I can't control often, and I feel pretty stressed a lot of the time—2 points
- A little stress can send me into a tailspin; I have no coping skills that really work for me—3 points
- I'm a walking stress ball, pretty much in a constant state of fight or flight—4 points

6. On average, how often do you move your body for at least thirty minutes a day, where you work up a sweat?
   - Daily—0 points
   - A few times a week—1 point
   - Once a week—2 points
   - A few times a month—3 points
   - Rarely or never—4 points

7. How much water do you drink each day?
   - 64 ounces (eight 8-ounce glasses) of water or more—0 points
   - Seven 8-ounce glasses of water—1 point
   - Six 8-ounce glasses of water—2 points
   - Five 8-ounce glasses of water—3 points
   - Four or fewer 8-ounce glasses of water—4 points

Scoring

Now it's time to take a look at your answers today and score yourself. Add up your points and write your total score here: _____

Progress Report:
I went from ___ total points on this quiz to ___ total points on this quiz in just 17 days.

0–7 points: You're mastering the "more of the good, less of the bad" philosophy! Keep it up and try to push yourself each day to head toward a 0 score.

8–14 points: You're doing well, and there's always room for improvement. Think of each day as its own challenge to move your score into the 0–7 category.

15–21 points: Your behavior is starting to reflect your desire to make changes in your health, and if you put forth a little more effort, you'll start to experience even more positive results.

22–28 points: Your current lifestyle isn't contributing to your overall health or weight loss goals, but you likely recognize the areas that need your immediate attention, and you have lots of opportunity to celebrate your incremental improvements. You've got this!

HOW YOU'RE FEELING INVENTORY

How have you been feeling overall from day to day? Let's reassess and see if things have shifted for you since you started.

Answer each question in this quiz honestly and thoughtfully. Give yourself a second to think about your average day and how you really feel.

1. Does your stomach feel or appear bloated, especially within an hour or so after eating?
   - Never/very rarely—0 points
   - Sometimes, after a big meal or after foods I know tend to cause gas—1 point
   - Fairly often, at least a couple times a week—2 points
   - A lot of the time—3 points
   - Most of the time/constantly—4 points

2. Do you experience digestive issues such as heartburn, gas, loose stool, constipation, nausea?
   - Never/very rarely—0 points
   - Sometimes, especially after I eat or drink specific foods or beverages—1 point
   - Fairly often, at least a couple times a week—2 points

- A lot of the time—3 points
- Daily or much of the time—4 points

3. What are your energy levels like?
   - I always have a good amount of energy to complete the tasks I want to, and I have some left over at the end of the day—0 points
   - I run out of steam if I push myself, but for the most part, I have enough energy to sustain me throughout the day—1 point
   - I have sinking spells from time to time, and need to rest during the day—2 points
   - I start to lose energy pretty early in the day, and I struggle to make it through to bedtime—3 points
   - I wake up tired, fight exhaustion all day, pretty much every day—4 points

4. Do you get headaches?
   - Never/very rarely—0 points
   - Sometimes, but usually because I didn't drink enough water—1 point
   - I notice my head hurting, like a dull pain, fairly often—2 points
   - I get debilitating headaches sometimes, and less serious ones often—3 points
   - Headaches have become such a part of my life that I practically put them in my schedule—4 points

5. Do you experience moodiness or mood swings?
   - Never/very rarely—0 points
   - Sometimes, but it's usually hormone-related—1 point
   - I am moody fairly often—2 points
   - My family hides behind the curtains because my mood swings so wildly a lot of the time—3 points
   - The least little thing will send me into a tirade . . . and for good reason! The world is driving me crazy!—4 points

6. Do you ever find yourself struggling with lack of motivation?
   - Never/very rarely—0 points
   - Sometimes, but it's usually because something threw me off—1 point
   - Fairly often I find it tough to get motivated to do what I want and need to do in a day—2 points
   - It takes a lot to get me motivated these days; I'd rather just pretend my to-do list is done already—3 points
   - Getting out of bed in the morning is a struggle—in fact, it's noon and I'm still in it right now—4 points

7. Do you ever have trouble focusing, paying attention, or remembering things?
   - Never/very rarely; I'm sharp as a tack—0 points
   - Occasionally I have a case of brain fog, but those are few and far between—1 point
   - I'm noticing this being a problem for me more lately (forgetting where I left my keys, feeling distracted and like I can't focus on the task at hand)—2 points
   - This happens so often that it scares me; my brain just won't hold information the way it used to—3 points
   - What's my name again? And what's this book I'm reading?—4 points

8. How many hours of sleep are you averaging per night?
   - 8+ hours—0 points
   - 7 hours—1 point
   - 6 hours—2 points
   - 5 hours—3 points
   - 4 or fewer hours—4 points

9. How often are you waking up per night?
   - Once my head hits the pillow, I'm out until it's time to wake up—0 points

- I might wake up once in a while to go to the bathroom, but it's rare and I can go right back to sleep—1 point
- I wake up occasionally, and when I do, I struggle to go back to sleep—2 points
- I wake up pretty often, and I have to read to fall back to sleep—3 points
- I'm up half the night, restless, unable to string together more than a couple hours of good sleep—4 points

Scoring

0–9 points: Overall, you're likely feeling good, and if there are areas that need improvement, you likely know what those areas are. You can use the tools in this book to feel your absolute best in all areas!

10–18 points: Like all of us, you likely have good days and bad days. Use this assessment as a way to know exactly where to put your energy as you read through this book and begin to implement the tools in your life.

19–27 points: There are probably a couple of areas of your well-being that are feeling off, but once you get focused on them, you will experience serious improvements. You'll soon have specific strategies for each category, and the power to feel better will be in your hands.

28–36 points: You might feel like you're struggling every day, but the great news is that you don't have to struggle anymore. Even improving one area of your overall wellness will have a powerful ripple effect on the rest of your health.

As we've talked about, goal-setting shouldn't just be about weight loss—you should have goals in other areas of your life such as:

- Reducing the effects of stress/boosting resilience
- Increasing mental acuity
- Improving sleep
- Increasing daily movement/flexibility and reducing injury risk

It's all about winning those key battles, and it's not a one-time thing. It's every day.

Progress Report:
I went from ____ total points on this quiz to _____ total points on this quiz in just 17 days.

What are some areas of your overall health that have improved already, as a result of the changes you've made using this plan?

_____

_____

_____

What are some areas of your overall health that you'd still like to work toward improving?

_____

_____

_____

If you have big goals, like losing a hundred pounds or getting off medications you've been on for a long time, it's easy to feel overwhelmed. But instead of focusing on the big end goal, turn your attention to how you're going to achieve it. Set smaller goals along the way, and get excited when you hit them. When you try to run uphill too fast, you fall on your face. You have to take it slowly, incrementally.

My dad was always great about giving me plenty of what he referred to as "atta-boys." Anytime I helped him with chores or did something he asked, he always gave me praise, and it made me feel good. Everyone likes praise. But as adults, we seldom have people around us giving us those "atta-boys" or "atta-girls" when we accomplish a goal. So we have to be sure to give ourselves the praise we need to keep on going.

If you were drinking ten soft drinks a day, and you got down to five, give yourself a big pat on the back. That's awesome progress. If you have lost two pounds, do a little happy dance, because you are two pounds closer to your goal. Acknowledging your progress is just as important as actually making the progress.

What are your specific, smaller goals that will help you achieve your overall goals?

_____

_____

_____

One pitfall to keep your eye out for is turning to unhealthy food, drugs, or alcohol to celebrate wins along the way. I know it can be tempting to run out and pick up your favorite pizza when you're excited, but clearly, that's a counterproductive choice. One of my guilty pleasures is ice cream. I have fond memories of sitting with my mom watching TV and eating ice cream together. But now she's not around to tell me not to eat directly from the carton, so I end up overindulging. So instead, if I've achieved a health goal or am celebrating the end of a long week, I choose something else, like one glass of wine with a 6-ounce filet.

Take a little time to think about the healthy ways you can celebrate your wins along the way so that you aren't tempted to engage in something that sabotages the very progress you're celebrating.

Healthy ways I can celebrate my progress are:

_____

_____

_____

Now that you have some ideas for rewarding yourself for all the goals you hit, big or small, put them into action! The more positive you are about the progress you're making, the more motivated you will feel to keep going. Take some pride in your hard work.

CONCLUSION

If you look back across time at the human body, not much has changed since the days of the caveman. We still have one heart, two lungs, two kidneys, and so on. Structurally speaking, we are largely the same as we were in the beginning. But do you know what has changed dramatically? Our environment. The world in which we now live is totally different from when we were hunters and gatherers. Unfortunately, our world today is rich with toxic pollutants—things like fast food or poor-quality food, work demands, long stretches of sitting at a computer, and, yes, even the air we breathe. We are being bombarded from all angles with new tools, new ideas, and new challenges. Our job is to adapt by choosing to control the controllable factors. When we do that, all of those toxic pollutants don't affect us nearly as much.

That's exactly what we've been working on together throughout this whole process: adapting. Modifying your lifestyle choices so that you can exist as the healthiest possible version of yourself in the real world. You're now choosing the foods that will fuel you and help you lose unnecessary fat. You're choosing to exercise your body, and to properly manage stress as it comes. You've built up a support system of people who are there for you, cheering you on and showing up when the going gets tough.

As you've likely realized, adapting in these ways and thus creating lasting change in our lives first requires that we get honest with ourselves about our habits, behavior, and why we do what we do. That's not always easy. But if you approach it in such a way that you give yourself grace, rather than guilt, it's easier.

Your story—your history—plays a big role in all of this. We've all been through painful times in our past. If you let it, that pain can have profound effects on your present. This is especially true if you choose to ignore it and pretend it isn't there. Had I gone into denial about the emotional upheaval I felt following my divorce and then the deaths of my mother and sister, well, I don't know what would have happened. But it wouldn't have ended well. Instead, I sought help, and I allowed myself to experience the sadness and the grief so that I could then move through it to the next phase of my life. Those will always be painful memories, but those memories don't have to haunt me, or cause me to make harmful choices. There's a real freedom in honoring our history, even the painful parts, but not letting it dictate our future.

As a doctor, I try to meet every patient exactly where they are, in whatever part of their life story they are currently experiencing. And then I try to help them write the next scene. And then the next, until they're living a healthy version of their lives. I hope you have been using the tools within these pages to create that for yourself.

So much of what you've accomplished here has to do with resiliency. You are able to bounce back from setbacks, to deal with stress as it comes, and to refuse to let life's potholes keep you from winning the key battles. You know that you are capable of making the healthiest choices, without getting caught up in an all-or-nothing mentality. Take a moment and see yourself for the resilient individual that you are.

Health, like life, is dynamic. It is ever-changing and evolving. That's great news, because it means every day provides you with a new opportunity to choose more of the good, and less of the bad. My sincere hope is that this book put more of the power over your life back into your hands, right where it belongs. You can always return to the parts of this book that resonate with you, and use it as a guide for everyday resiliency.

Know that my team and I are here to support you every step of the way. You can join the private Facebook page we have set up, the 17 Day Challenge. Just visit: drmikediet.com. I often do live sessions where you can ask your questions and I'll answer them. But more important, there you will find a community that will accept and support you from day one. I hope you'll join.

Thank you for trusting me with helping you reach your goals. I wish you more of the good in your life, now and in the future.

RECIPES

1. GREEN OMEGA SMOOTHIE

This smoothie packs a nutritious punch and is sure to fill you up with plenty of healthy fiber. And it tastes fantastic too. A great way to start your day.

Phase: Scrub, Soak Up, Stabilize

Serves: 1

- 2 cups coconut water
- 1 cup strawberries (fresh or frozen)
- 2 cups leafy greens (spinach, kale, supergreens mix)
- ¼ avocado
- 1 tablespoon ground flax or chia seeds
- 3 tablespoons hemp seeds
- A few ice cubes (optional)

Place all the ingredients in your blender and blend until smooth.

Notes:

This is a meal replacement smoothie. Feel free to experiment with amounts to find the best flavor and consistency for your taste!

Go for the greens! This tasty sauté will give you the phytonutrients your body really wants. The lemon and garlic combination goes perfectly with any leafy greens you choose.

Phase: Scrub, Soak Up, Stabilize
Serves: 1 to 2

1 (5- to 6-ounce) bag leafy greens (mixed or just one type), cut and washed

1 tablespoon oil (avocado oil, coconut oil, extra-virgin olive oil)

Dash of sea salt

2 garlic cloves, minced

Squeeze of lemon (optional)

Pinch of black pepper (optional)

1. Open the bag of leafy greens and set aside.
2. Heat a large sauté pan over medium-high heat and add the oil.
3. Add the greens to the pan with a dash of salt and sauté for 30 seconds.
4. Add the garlic and cover the pan with a lid for 1 minute, until the greens are tender and bright green.
5. Remove the lid and sauté for another 3 minutes or until al dente. Add lemon juice and pepper, if using.

Notes:

- Keeping the lid on the pan at the start of cooking utilizes steam and moisture to cook the greens, cutting back on the use of oil, and prevents burning. You may have to keep your lid on longer than a minute, depending on the greens you use.
- You can use one type of green like kale or spinach or buy a pack that contains mixed greens.

3. QUICK CELERY AND PARSLEY DETOX SALAD

The flavors in this salad go together like a beautiful piece of music. One ingredient complements the next to create a delightful medley. Plus, it has a nice crunch!

Phase: Scrub, Soak Up, Stabilize

Serves: 2

7 small to medium stalks celery

⅓ cup flat-leaf parsley

¼ cup fresh pomegranate seeds

Pinch of sea salt

Pinch of cracked black pepper (optional)

Drizzle of olive oil

Squeeze of lemon juice

1. Peel off the excess fibrous threads and finely chop the celery on the diagonal.
2. Finely chop the parsley.
3. Combine the celery, parsley, and pomegranate seeds in a large mixing bowl, and toss together. Add the salt, pepper (if using), oil, and lemon juice.

4. GARLICKY TUSCAN BEANS AND SWISS GREENS

This dish reminds me of a side dish at Thanksgiving dinner. Bursting with flavor as well as fiber, this is a whole meal all by itself.

Phase: Scrub, Soak Up, Stabilize

Serves: 2

2 heaping cups (packed) chard

2 tablespoons olive oil

½ onion, chopped

5 garlic cloves, minced

1 stalk celery, diced

1 carrot, diced

1½ cups cannellini beans

1 ounce sun-dried tomatoes

Pinch of red pepper flakes

Have on hand (optional):

Lemon wedges

Sea salt and black pepper

3 tablespoons chopped fresh parsley

1 teaspoon chopped fresh oregano

Olive oil to drizzle

1. Rinse and dry the chard and chop.
2. Heat the 2 tablespoons oil in a sauté pan and add the onion, garlic, celery, and carrot. Sweat with the lid on the pan until they are al dente and fragrant.
3. Add the cannellini beans and sun-dried tomatoes, and cook uncovered for another 5 minutes.
4. Add the chard, red pepper flakes, and an extra dash of oil (if needed), and cook for a few more minutes with the lid back on until the chard is wilted and the dish is properly mixed together. Be careful not to mash the beans.
5. Finish to taste, if desired, with a squeeze of lemon, salt, pepper, parsley, and oregano.

5. QUICK SALMON SALAD

Who knew canned salmon could taste so good? This salad takes no time to make and is sure to leave you feeling super satisfied.

Phase: Soak Up, Stabilize

Serves: 2

1 (6-ounce) can wild salmon

½ cup finely chopped celery

1 teaspoon chopped capers

¼ cup minced shallots

3 tablespoons Vegenaise (made with avocado oil)

1 tablespoon chopped fresh dill

1 teaspoon lemon juice

Pinch of salt (optional)

1. Put the salmon in a bowl and break it up with a fork.
2. Add the remaining ingredients to the salmon, and combine well.
3. Add salt and additional seasoning to taste, if desired.

Notes:

This can be served in lettuce cups, using butter lettuce, green leaf, or romaine. Or serve on top of whole grain crispbreads, flax crackers, or whole grain sprouted bread.

Your whole house will smell amazing while this is heating up. This warm, comforting veggie bake is a crowd pleaser, so make it for the whole family or invite some friends over!

Phase: Scrub, Soak Up, Stabilize

Serves: 4

Avocado oil cooking spray

2 teaspoons Italian seasoning *

2 tablespoons olive oil (or more as needed)

3 garlic cloves, minced

1 head broccoli, chopped into florets

1 head cauliflower, chopped into florets

1 pound brussels sprouts, cut in half

1 yellow bell pepper, chopped

½ red onion, chopped

1 cup cherry tomatoes, sliced

Sea salt and black pepper to taste

*Oregano, basil, parsley, thyme, garlic, red pepper—these can be used dried or fresh; one or more may be omitted and you'll still have plenty of seasoning.

1. Preheat the oven to 450°F. Line a large baking sheet with parchment paper sprayed lightly with the avocado oil cooking spray. Set aside.
2. In a large mixing bowl, whisk the Italian seasoning and olive oil. Add the garlic, broccoli, cauliflower, brussels sprouts, bell pepper, and onion, and combine until the oil is evenly distributed. If needed, you can add up to another tablespoon of olive oil.
3. Spread the vegetable mixture in a single layer on the baking sheet.
4. Bake for 20 minutes. Stir the veggies and add the cherry tomatoes, then bake for another 15 minutes. Season with salt and pepper.

7. EASY CREAMY TOMATO SOUP

The coconut milk adds just a touch of sweetness to this classic soup recipe. Perfect for a chilly evening, or anytime a warm bowl of soup is just what the doctor ordered.

Phase: Scrub, Soak Up, Stabilize

Serves: 4

½ tablespoon olive oil

2 garlic cloves, minced

1 sweet onion, chopped

1 (28-ounce) can whole peeled tomatoes

1½ cups water

1 teaspoon Italian seasoning

½ teaspoon salt or more to taste

1 (13.5-ounce) can coconut milk

Black pepper to taste

Cayenne pepper (optional)

1. Heat the oil in a large saucepan over medium heat.
2. Add the garlic and onion, and cook for 5 minutes.
3. Add the tomatoes, water, Italian seasoning, and salt, and gently mash the tomatoes with a wooden spoon.
4. Bring to a boil, then reduce the heat and simmer for 10 minutes.
5. Stir in the coconut milk, then remove from the heat and let cool for 5 minutes.
6. Transfer the mixture to a blender and blend until smooth.
7. Season to taste and serve.

Notes:
- You can use any other onion if there are no sweet onions available.
- Choose light coconut milk in order to reduce calories and fat grams.

This salad is bright, crisp, and crunchy. Make a couple servings and save some for tomorrow, when you're sure to be craving it again.

Phase: Scrub, Soak Up, Stabilize

Serves: 2 to 4

Snap Pea Salad

2 cups sugar snap peas

¼ cup sliced red onion

½ cup diced cucumber

5 mint leaves, coarsely chopped

Salt and black pepper to taste

1. Wash the peas, then trim off the stems and remove the strings from the pods. Cut the peas in half on the diagonal.
2. Combine the peas, onion, cucumber, and mint in a bowl and toss. Season with salt and pepper to taste. Add 5-Minute Dressing and toss again.

5-Minute Dressing

1½ tablespoons honey

2 teaspoons Dijon mustard

1 small garlic clove, finely minced

¼ cup balsamic vinegar

2 tablespoons chopped fresh herbs (dill, thyme, oregano, chives, or whatever's on hand)

¼ teaspoon fine sea salt

⅓ cup extra-virgin olive oil

1. In a small mixing bowl, whisk together all the ingredients except for the oil. When well-mixed, add the oil and whisk thoroughly to combine.
2. Use as much as desired for the salad, and store the rest in an airtight glass container in the refrigerator for up to 1 week. Double the recipe to make extra if preferred.

I'm willing to bet you've never had coleslaw quite like this one. The sesame dressing adds a unique flavor profile, and you can really make it your own with the optional ingredients.

Phase: Soak Up, Stabilize

Serves: 4

Rainbow Coleslaw

¼ cup thinly sliced green onions	1 (16-ounce) bag tricolor shredded cabbage/coleslaw
¼ cup cilantro, chopped	1 cup shredded carrots

1. Combine the green onions, cilantro, cabbage, and carrots in a large bowl and toss.
2. Add the dressing and toss again.

Sesame Dressing

½ teaspoon minced fresh ginger	sesame oil (be sure it's toasted)
½ teaspoon minced garlic	1 tablespoon avocado oil
1½ tablespoons toasted	1 tablespoon rice vinegar

Whisk all the ingredients together. Pour over the slaw and toss.

Notes:

Add any combination of the following to make the salad a complete meal: ½ cup sliced bell peppers; ⅓ cup toasted sliced almonds; ⅓ cup toasted chopped cashews or peanuts; 4 ounces of grilled chicken breast, shrimp, grilled salmon, grilled steak, or grilled tempeh.

These tartines are like little slices of heaven. With lots of options, you can tailor them to your own taste.

Phase: Scrub, Soak Up, Stabilize (depending on choices)
Serves: 1

2 large or 4 medium crisp-breads (oat, rye, seeds, flax)

Spread of choice (enough for a thin layer on each crispbread):

Cashew cream cheese

Almond spreadable cheese

Avocado

Simple Avocado Salad (page 183)

Protein of choice (up to 4 ounces divided among crispbreads):

Cooked chicken breast

Smoked salmon

Mashed beans

Hummus

Hard-boiled eggs, sliced

Veggie toppings of choice (enough to heap on each crispbread):

Baby tomatoes

Cucumber

Sprouts

Microgreens

Arugula

Parsley

Lay out each crispbread cracker and apply your desired toppings. Keep as open-faced tartines.

Notes:

A crispbread is a large, flat, dry cracker made from rye flour; there are also gluten-free versions made with oats and/or seeds.

This is one of those soups you'll want to enjoy again and again. It tastes even better the next day—perfect for easy meal prep on busy nights. Make a big batch on Sunday and enjoy it every day throughout the week!

Phase: Soak Up, Stabilize

Serves: 4 to 6

6 cups vegetable broth

2 medium carrots, chopped

½ onion, finely chopped

3 garlic cloves, minced

½ cup tomatoes (from can/jar/ carton), diced

1 (15-ounce) can chickpeas

2 teaspoons Italian seasoning

¼ teaspoon paprika

1 box (8 ounces) chickpea fusilli pasta

Lemon juice to taste

Salt and black pepper to taste

1. Add ⅓ cup of the vegetable broth to a stockpot and bring to a boil.
2. Turn down to medium heat and add the carrots, onion, and garlic. Cook until the onion is translucent and carrots are tender.
3. Add the remaining broth, the tomatoes, chickpeas, Italian seasoning, and paprika, and cook for 5 minutes.
4. Pour half of the mixture into a blender and blend gently. Pour the puree back into the stockpot and mix with the remaining soup.
5. Add the chickpea pasta and cook for 8 minutes, until al dente.
6. Serve with a squeeze of lemon and added salt and pepper, if preferred.

12. BAKED SWEET POTATO FRIES

Fries on a diet? Oh yes I did! Satisfy your desire for the salty favorites, but without the trans fat.

Phase: Soak Up, Stabilize

Serves: 2 to 3

2 large sweet potatoes

1 tablespoon tapioca flour or arrowroot flour

¼ teaspoon fine sea salt

2 tablespoons olive oil or coconut oil (melted)

Black pepper, cayenne pepper, garlic powder, or any other seasoning (optional)

1. Preheat the oven to 425°F with one rack in the lower third of the oven and the other in the top third at least 6 inches from the heat source.
2. Line two large rimmed baking sheets with parchment paper.
3. Peel the sweet potatoes and cut them into fry-shaped pieces about ¼ inch wide and ¼ inch thick.
4. Toss the sweet potatoes in a bowl with the flour and salt until evenly coated.
5. Divide the uncooked fries between the baking sheets. Arrange the fries in a single layer, being careful not to crowd them.
6. Drizzle the oil over the fries, using 1 tablespoon for each sheet.
7. Bake for 15 minutes. Flip the fries and bake for 15 minutes longer.
8. Enjoy the fries as is, or season with additional salt, pepper, cayenne, garlic powder, or whatever you prefer!

Notes:

If you don't have tapioca flour or arrowroot flour, you can use cornstarch—but the tapioca and arrowroot are definitely healthier options!

13. CHIPOTLE FISH TACOS

Though the typical restaurant version of fish tacos includes fried fish, this version is made with sautéed whitefish, and I'd argue it's even tastier than what you can get in a restaurant. Plus, of course, it's far healthier.

Phase: Scrub, Soak Up, Stabilize

Serves: 3 to 4

3 tablespoons lime juice

1 tablespoon chipotle powder

3 garlic cloves, minced

½ tablespoon canned jalapeño, chopped

2 tablespoons olive oil, plus 1 tablespoon for sautéing

⅓ cup cilantro, chopped, plus more to garnish

1 pound whitefish (tilapia, snapper, or cod)

4 or more lettuce cups (butter lettuce, romaine, or iceberg)

1. Mix together the lime juice, chipotle, garlic, jalapeño, the 2 tablespoons oil, and the cilantro. Pour over the fish and marinate for 30 minutes.
2. Lightly coat a skillet with oil and cook the fish over high heat, 2 to 3 minutes on each side.
3. Add the fish to the prepared lettuce cups and top with extra lettuce and cilantro. Remember, cilantro has some detoxifying benefits, so pile it on!

14. FALL ANY THYME WILD RICE PILAF

This pilaf makes a hearty meal with great texture. Onion, garlic, and fragrant herbs make it rich and flavorful.

Phase: Stabilize

Serves: 2

1¾ cups broth (chicken or vegetable)

1 cup wild rice blend

1½ tablespoons olive oil

3 garlic cloves, chopped

Several sprigs of fresh sage, chopped

1 small onion, chopped

4 ounces cremini mushrooms, chopped

1 tablespoon chopped fresh thyme

1 tablespoon chopped fresh oregano

1. In a stockpot, combine the broth and rice and bring to a boil. Turn down to a medium simmer and cook for 35 to 45 minutes with the lid on. Check periodically, and turn off when the rice has absorbed all the water.
2. In a separate sauté pan, heat 1 tablespoon of the oil. Add the garlic and sage, and sauté until you start to smell the aromatic sage.
3. Add the onion and sauté for another minute.
4. Add the mushrooms, thyme, and oregano and the remaining ½ tablespoon oil to the sauté pan. Cook for 5 to 10 minutes, until the mushrooms are tender and brown on one side.
5. Add the mushroom mixture to the rice pilaf and combine evenly.

Notes:

This dish can be topped with 4 ounces of meat such as chicken, or with navy beans for a plant-based protein punch.

The healthy fat found in avocado makes this easy salad one that really sticks to your ribs. And it's the perfect vehicle for fresh, detoxifying herbs.

Phase: Scrub, Soak Up, Stabilize

Serves: 1 to 2

1 heaping cup chopped avocado

⅓ cup chopped red onion

⅓ cup chopped cucumber

⅓ cup shredded carrots

2 tablespoons finely chopped

parsley or cilantro

1½ tablespoons olive oil

1 tablespoon lemon juice

Sea salt

1. Place the avocado, onion, cucumber, carrots, and parsley in a bowl and combine using a large spoon or spatula.
2. Drizzle with oil and lemon juice, and add salt to taste. Enjoy!

16. ABC PUDDING

This might sound like an odd combination of ingredients, but trust me when I tell you it all works together beautifully. Before long, ABC Pudding will be your go-to dessert. If you have kids, let them give it a try. They might just be requesting it every day!

Phase: Soak Up, Stabilize

Serves: 3 to 4

1 avocado, very ripe

2 large bananas, very ripe

2 tablespoons cocoa powder, unsweetened

1. Combine all three ingredients in a blender or mini food processor and blend until smooth.
2. Chill in the refrigerator for at least 1 hour before serving. This step is a must to reach the desired pudding texture and flavor!

Notes:

- While this tastes like a decadent dessert, it does not need any added sweetener as long as your bananas are very ripe. If you don't have the ripest bananas or just want a touch more sweetness, you can add up to 1 tablespoon of honey.
- Try adding a pinch of cinnamon or nutmeg and/or ½ teaspoon of vanilla extract for extra flavor. You can also top with additional ingredients like berries or slivered almonds.
- Freeze the bananas ahead of time before blending for optimal texture and less chilling time.

17. KALE CRUNCHIES

Sometimes we all just need to munch on something, and kale crunchies are the perfect solution. Who needs potato chips when you've got these?

Phase: Scrub, Soak Up, Stabilize

Serves: 3 to 4

1 bunch kale

2 tablespoons avocado oil

1 teaspoon garlic powder

½ teaspoon cumin

1 teaspoon sea salt

1. Preheat the oven to 275°F.
2. Wash and dry the kale. Remove the ribs and rip or cut it into 1- to 2-inch pieces.
3. In a large bowl, pour the oil over the kale and mix with your hands until it is lightly covered.
4. Add the garlic, cumin, and salt, and continue mixing to coat evenly.
5. Line a baking sheet with parchment paper and spread the kale on it, making sure the pieces don't overlap too much to ensure they all get crispy.
6. Bake for 20 minutes or until crispy.

Notes:

It's key that the kale not be wet when you put it in the oven. After washing kale, let it dry entirely or put it through a salad spinner to remove all moisture. You can also purchase bagged kale that is prewashed and nice and dry—and if it's already in small pieces, all you have to do is remove the ribs.

18. BANANA BERRY "ICE CREAM"

Step away from the ice cream aisle; you don't need all that sugar! Especially when this fruity "ice cream" is sure to satisfy your sweet tooth.

Phase: Soak Up, Stabilize

Serves: 4

4 bananas, very ripe   2 cups sliced frozen strawberries

1. Peel the bananas and slice into ½-inch pieces. Freeze overnight.
2. Place the frozen banana slices and strawberry slices in a food processor or powerful blender. Puree the mixture, scraping down the container when needed. Keep blending until smooth.
3. Serve immediately for soft-serve ice cream consistency; if you prefer harder ice cream, place it in a freezer container and freeze for at least 1 hour before serving.

19. LEMON-CUCUMBER-MINT DETOX AID

Sip on this this ultra-hydrating, refreshing drink first thing in the morning or in the middle of the afternoon for a little pick-me-up. Drink to your health!

Phase: Scrub, Soak Up, Stabilize

Serves: 2

½ cucumber

6 mint leaves

1 large lemon

1½ liters filtered water

1. Rinse the cucumber and mint. Remove the mint leaves from the stems.
2. Cut the cucumber and lemon into thin slices
3. Pour the water into a pitcher or a 64-ounce large-mouth mason jar. Stir in the cucumber, mint leaves, and lemon. Chill in the refrigerator.
4. Drink half of it early in the morning and the rest in the second part of the day. This cleansing drink will aid weight loss, metabolism, digestion, and energy especially during the Scrub phase.

20. SOAK IT UP SEED BREAD

Even the least-talented bakers can make this simple and tasty seed bread. It's great to have on hand for a quick breakfast or snack.

Phase: Soak Up, Stabilize

Serves: About 12 (makes 1 loaf)

1 cup sunflower seeds

½ cup flaxseeds

¼ cup chia seeds

1½ cups rolled oats

3 tablespoons psyllium seed-husk powder

1 teaspoon sea salt

1½ cups filtered water

3 tablespoons coconut oil, melted

1 tablespoon maple syrup

1. In a large bowl, combine all of the dry ingredients.
2. In a separate small bowl, mix the water, oil, and maple syrup.
3. Add the wet ingredients to the dry ingredients and mix well until everything is combined and the dough is thick. If it's too thick to work with (meaning, it's not easy to knead), add a teaspoon of water and mix again.
4. Line a loaf pan with parchment, keeping the edges of the parchment higher than the sides of the pan. Pour the mixture in and smooth out the top. Let sit overnight.
5. Preheat the oven to 350°F.
6. Bake the loaf for 20 minutes.
7. Remove the loaf from the pan by pulling up the sides of the parchment. Place it upside down directly on the oven rack and bake for another 40 minutes.
8. Let it cool completely before slicing.

21. CHERRY SOAK POPS

Have a hankering for an ice pop? Coming right up! These frozen cherry treats are sweet, satisfying, and so much fun.

Phase: Soak Up, Stabilize

Serves: 6

1 cup cherries, fresh or frozen

¼ cup coconut water

¼ cup coconut milk

1 tablespoon chia seeds

1. Mix all the ingredients in a high-powered blender.
2. Pour the mixture into ice pop molds and add sticks.
3. Place in the freezer and freeze at least 8 hours, preferably overnight, before eating.

Notes:

If you're not in the Scrub phase, you could boost the sweetness with up to 2 teaspoons of maple syrup or 2 teaspoons of monk fruit.

Acorn squash is one of my favorite types of squash. It's loaded with fiber and vitamin C, and it tastes fantastic on its own, but when combined with the ingredients in this recipe, it's off-the-charts delicious.

Phase: Scrub, Soak Up, Stabilize

Serves: 4

2 acorn squash

6 large shallots

½ teaspoon garlic powder

1 teaspoon smoked paprika

1 teaspoon dried oregano

Pinch of dried sage

Dash of sea salt

Dash of black pepper

⅓ cup plus 2 tablespoons olive oil

2 teaspoons apple cider vinegar

1. Preheat the oven to 425°F.
2. Using a sharp knife, cut the squash in half and scoop out the seeds. Then cut each half into 8 wedges.
3. Trim the shallots and remove the outer skin.
4. Place the squash and shallots together on a baking tray and season with the garlic powder, paprika, oregano, sage, salt, and pepper. Then drizzle evenly with the 2 tablespoons oil.
5. Roast for 30 to 40 minutes, turning the shallots once halfway through.
6. In a bowl, combine the ⅓ cup oil and the apple cider vinegar, seasoning with salt and pepper to taste. Drizzle over the roasted squash and shallots and serve.

23. STEAK SALAD WITH NO-OIL LEMON DRESSING

Sometimes you just want to sit down and devour a steak. At least, I do. When you aren't eating red meat on a regular basis, it becomes much more of a delicacy. This salad is an excellent way to enjoy a steak. And the dressing is oil-free since the steak has enough fat already. Dig in!

Phase: Stabilize

Serves: 2

Steak Salad

½ pound flank steak

Salt and black pepper to taste

Avocado oil spray

4 cups mixed leafy greens

½ cup cherry tomatoes

1. Season the steak with salt and pepper.
2. Heat a grill or pan to medium-high and spray with a thin layer of oil. Grill the steak for 4 to 6 minutes on each side.
3. Cut the steak into slices and arrange over the leafy greens and tomatoes. Drizzle with lemon dressing.

No-Oil Lemon Dressing

3 tablespoons filtered water

3 tablespoons apple cider vinegar

3 tablespoons lemon juice

2 garlic cloves, minced

¼ teaspoon onion salt

1 teaspoon dried oregano

1 teaspoon dried tarragon

Whisk all the ingredients together. Pour over the steak salad.

Notes:

You can replace the filtered water with oil for a slightly richer dressing.

Your local coffee shop's got nothing on this little cup of bliss. It's rich, sweet, and oh-so-healthy.

Phase: Stabilize

Serves: 1

½ teaspoon matcha powder

½ cup filtered water, hot (not boiling)

Honey to taste

Ginger to taste, dried or fresh

½ cup unsweetened coconut milk, warm

1. Whisk the matcha with about ¼ cup water until all lumps dissolve. You can use a wire whisk, a bamboo whisk, or a frother wand.
2. Once it's smooth, add the honey and ginger and whisk until well combined.
3. Pour in the remaining water and the coconut milk. Whisk until you reach the desired consistency. Enjoy right away.

25. OVERNIGHT CHIA PUDDING

If you've ever had overnight oats, this is a similar concept but with chia seeds. It's sure to be a fan favorite—sweet, super filling, and a great way to start the day.

Phase: Scrub, Soak Up, Stabilize

Serves: 2

1 cup canned light coconut milk

1 tablespoon maple syrup

⅓ cup chia seeds

1 teaspoon vanilla extract

½ cup berries

1. Add the coconut milk, maple syrup, chia seeds, and vanilla to a mixing bowl and whisk together.
2. Cover and refrigerate overnight.
3. When ready to eat, top with the berries.

Notes:

- You can use stevia or monk fruit instead of maple syrup—add a small amount of sweetener at a time and adjust according to your taste preference.
- You can substitute unsweetened cashew milk, hazelnut milk, or your dairy-free milk of choice for the coconut milk. Almond milk is also an option, although the pudding will be less thick.

This protein-packed breakfast is perfect for the whole family. The shredded coconut gives it a tropical twist.

Phase: Stabilize

Serves: 1

½ cup water

2 tablespoons almond flour

½ tablespoon shredded coconut

2 tablespoons hemp seeds

½ teaspoon monk fruit*

1 tablespoon peanut butter, natural and creamy

½ teaspoon vanilla extract

Pinch of cinnamon

¼ cup berries or favorite fruit (optional)

*Monk fruit is available at most health food markets such as Whole Foods, as well as online at retailers like Amazon. Many conventional grocery stores are also starting to carry it. However, be aware that the less-processed brands are usually found online and in health food stores.

1. Blend the water, almond flour, coconut, hemp seeds, and monk fruit in a microwave-safe bowl.
2. Microwave on high for 1 minute 30 seconds.
3. Immediately stir in the peanut butter, vanilla, and cinnamon.
4. Top with berries or your favorite fruit as desired.

Notes:

- In place of monk fruit, you can substitute an equal amount of stevia or ½ tablespoon of maple syrup. You can also drizzle a touch of extra sweetener on top of the porridge after removing it from the microwave.
- For cocoa-flavored porridge, add 1 teaspoon of cocoa powder.
- You can use any other nut or seed butter in place of peanut butter.

27. EGG MUFFINS

Who needs drive-thru breakfast sandwiches when you can have these delightful, nutrient-rich egg muffins? These little babies are great for breakfast, lunch, or dinner.

Phase: Soak Up, Stabilize

Serves: 6

2 teaspoons avocado oil

½ cup chopped red or green bell peppers

½ cup chopped yellow onion

1 cup spinach, chopped

½ cup sliced mushrooms

1 garlic clove, minced

¼ teaspoon sea salt

2 whole eggs

2 egg whites

1. Preheat the oven to 350°F. Grease the cups of a six-muffin pan or line with paper liners, preferably parchment paper.
2. Heat a large nonstick skillet over medium heat. Add the oil, bell peppers, and onion. Sauté for 5 minutes.
3. Add the spinach, mushrooms, and garlic and cook for an additional 2 minutes. Finish with the salt.
4. Whisk the whole eggs and egg whites together, then combine with the veggies.
5. Pour the egg and veggie mixture evenly into the muffin pan. Bake for 18 to 20 minutes.

Notes:

These are great to refrigerate for up to 4 days, or you can even freeze them. Reheat in the toaster oven or microwave for a ready-to-go breakfast.

28. AVOCADO SMOKED SALMON WRAP

These are the simplest, fastest-to-prepare wraps you've ever had. Loaded with healthy fats, they're sure to fill you up too!

Phase: Scrub, Soak Up, Stabilize

Serves: 1

½ medium avocado

2 ounces smoked salmon

Sea salt and black pepper to taste

1. Slice the avocado. Wrap each slice in smoked salmon.
2. Season with salt and pepper.

Notes:

Add to a bed of arugula or spinach, or put on top of seed bread. Alternatively, replace the avocado with a cashew- or almond-based cheese spread (a good one is Miyoko's).

29. ALMOND FLOUR PANCAKES

Sometimes you just want to eat pancakes. I get it! The next time you've got the hankering, whip up this healthy version instead of a store-bought mix. You'll be so glad you did!

Phase: Soak Up, Stabilize

Serves: 1

⅔ cup almond flour	½ tablespoon almond milk
⅓ teaspoon baking powder	2 teaspoons avocado oil
½ large egg	Pinch of sea salt
1 teaspoon monk fruit	½ cup berries (optional)

1. Whisk together the almond flour, baking powder, egg, monk fruit, almond milk, oil, and salt.
2. Heat a greased skillet over medium-low heat.
3. Pour the batter into the skillet, no more than ⅛ cup at a time. Cook each side for 4 minutes or until the pancake is browned.
4. Top with berries, if desired.

Notes:

- For a little sweetness, top with 1 teaspoon of 100% fruit jam, 1 teaspoon of maple syrup or coconut syrup, or liquid monk fruit to taste. Additionally, you can spread pancakes with up to 1 tablespoon of nut butter or sprinkle with 2 tablespoons of sliced almonds.
- Feel free to add a pinch or two of cinnamon and/or nutmeg to the batter for increased flavor and antioxidants!
- To yield more pancakes, double the recipe.

So many options, so little time! You can make your sweet potato toast just the way you like it—sweet or savory. And now that you've used sweet potato slices instead of bread to make toast, you'll never want to go back.

Phase: Scrub, Soak Up, Stabilize

Serves: 1

½ very large sweet potato or yam (larger is easier to slice)

¼ avocado

1 teaspoon pesto sauce

1 tablespoon nut butter (your choice)

1 teaspoon fruit jam (100% fruit)

½ cup berries

1 hard-boiled egg

½ banana, sliced

2 tablespoons seeds (sunflower, pumpkin, sesame, or your choice)

1. Trim the ends off the sweet potato and lay it on its side on a cutting board. Use a large knife to slice it lengthwise into ¼-inch slices.
2. Put the sweet potato slices into the toaster oven, set to 400°F, and toast until they are fork-tender but not soft. You may need to toast a third time. If you do not have a toaster, set your oven to broil and bake on a sheet for 4 to 6 minutes per side.
3. Allow the sweet potatoes to cool slightly on a wire rack before adding the toppings to make sure they don't get soggy.
4. Place the toasted sweet potato on a plate and add your choice of toppings.

Notes:

Option 1: Avocado, pesto, and seeds

Option 2: Avocado, hard-boiled egg, sea salt and pepper to taste

Option 3: Nut butter with either banana slices, berries, or jam

Option 4: Any combination from your ingredient list—there are so many options!

31. BAKED MUSTARD CHICKEN

If you've never used mustard when baking chicken, you've been missing out. It really helps the chicken stay moist, and it tastes amazing, especially with this specific combination of spices. It's a great weeknight meal that everyone in your household will enjoy!

Phase: Stabilize

Serves: 4

½ cup whole grain mustard

1 ounce lemon juice

2 garlic cloves, minced

1 teaspoon dried tarragon

½ teaspoon smoked paprika

½ teaspoon black pepper

¼ teaspoon salt (fine sea salt or kosher)

1 pound boneless, skinless chicken breasts

1 cucumber (any kind)

2 tomatoes (preferably Roma, or whatever available)

1. Preheat the oven to 400°F.
2. Combine the mustard, lemon juice, garlic, tarragon, paprika, pepper, and salt in a large bowl and mix well.
3. Add the chicken and mix into the sauce, making sure it is coated well.
4. Place the chicken and sauce in a large baking dish and cover with parchment paper. Bake for 25 to 30 minutes, until the chicken is cooked through.
5. Remove the chicken from the oven and let it rest, still covered, for 10 minutes before serving.
6. Chop the cucumber and tomatoes, and serve alongside chicken.

Notes:

- To maximize flavor and tenderness, marinate the chicken in the sauce for at least 30 minutes and up to 2 hours. Also, use a poultry thermometer when baking to check for internal temperature; once it reaches 165°F it is ready to come out (chicken breast tends to dry out if overcooked).
- You can substitute 1 to 2 tablespoons of fresh tarragon for the dried tarragon if you have it available.

Make this dish the night before and take it to work the next day, or just whip it up and eat it right away. It is fiber-rich and so tasty.

Phase: Scrub, Soak Up, Stabilize

Serves: 2

1 (15-ounce) can or carton black beans

½ cup chopped red bell pepper

2 tablespoons chopped red onion

½ avocado, chopped

1½ tablespoons lime juice

⅛ teaspoon chili powder

⅛ teaspoon cumin powder

Sea salt to taste

1 tablespoon cilantro, chopped in or as garnish

1. In a medium mixing bowl, combine the black beans, bell pepper, onion, and avocado.
2. Place the lime juice, chili powder, cumin, and salt in a mason jar. Add cilantro if desired (or save for garnish). Seal with a lid and shake until combined.
3. Pour the dressing over the black bean mixture and stir until evenly covered.
4. Serve immediately or refrigerate overnight to marinate the flavor.

Notes:

Garnish with extra cilantro for even more phytonutrients.

If you love curry, this is a wonderful alternative to the less-than-healthy types you might find at restaurants or in a takeout box. It has all the right flavors and all kinds of plant-based power.

Phase: Soak Up, Stabilize

Serves: 2

2 cups cauliflower florets

8 ounces tempeh

¼ cup low-sodium soy sauce or tamari sauce

1 tablespoon rice wine vinegar

1 teaspoon sesame oil

1 garlic clove, minced

1 tablespoon avocado oil

½ white onion

1 teaspoon minced fresh ginger

2½ teaspoons mild curry powder

¼ teaspoon turmeric

¼ teaspoon coriander

½ (13.5–ounce) can light coconut milk

½ (15-ounce) can or carton white beans

Squeeze of lime

1. Steam the cauliflower. (A quick microwave technique: Place the florets in a microwave-safe bowl with just enough water to cover the bottom, about 2 tablespoons, and cover with a plate. Microwave for 3 to 4 minutes, then let the cauliflower sit for 1 minute before removing from the microwave. Remove the plate—careful, the trapped steam will be hot—and let sit.)

2. Cut the tempeh into large cubes and marinate for 10 to 20 minutes in a mixture of the soy sauce, rice wine vinegar, ½ teaspoon of the sesame oil, and the garlic.

3. In a medium pan, use the remaining ½ teaspoon sesame oil to sauté the tempeh over medium heat until golden brown and crispy.

4. In a separate large pan, heat the avocado oil over medium-low heat. Add the onion and stir for 3 to 5 minutes until it softens and is translucent. Add the ginger, curry powder, turmeric, and coriander, then cook and stir for 2 minutes.

5. Add the coconut milk and bring to a simmer. Reduce the heat to low and simmer for 3 to 5 minutes, until slightly thickened. Add the beans, tempeh, and cauliflower, mixing them in evenly, and simmer for an additional 2 to 3 minutes. Squeeze a lime over the top.

Notes:

You can omit either the tempeh or the white beans; if so, increase cauliflower by 1 cup.

34. CHICKPEA SALAD

Chickpeas, also known as garbanzo beans, are a great meat replacement ingredient thanks to their protein content. Often used in Mediterranean-style meals, they go together really well with olive oil, red onions, and tomatoes, all of which are in this dish. The lemon juice adds a real brightness to the flavors.

Phase: Stabilize

Serves: 4

2 cups diced cucumbers

1 cup diced tomato

⅓ cup diced red onion

2 tablespoons lemon juice

½ tablespoon minced fresh parsley

1 tablespoon extra-virgin olive oil

½ teaspoon kosher salt

Cracked black pepper to taste

1 (15-ounce) can or carton garbanzo beans (rinsed and drained)

2 ounces low-fat mozzarella cheese, cubed, or fat-free crumbled feta to taste

Combine all the ingredients and toss. Enjoy!

Notes:

- Try adding additional veggies like bell peppers and tomatoes (½ cup each).
- You can also add half an avocado, cubed.
- If you opt for the feta cheese, reduce the amount of kosher salt to only a pinch or two. Athenos makes a tasty crumbled feta cheese that would work well.
- This is hearty enough to eat on its own; you can also serve it with flaxseed crackers.
- This recipe is even more flavorful when it marinates in the refrigerator overnight, or as leftovers the next day.

35. QUINOA TABOULI WITH SALMON

This is yet another fantastic way to dress up canned salmon for a quick, easy, and nutrient-dense meal. I love quinoa because it's so versatile, and it's a great source of vitamins and minerals including B vitamins and magnesium.

Phase: Scrub, Soak Up, Stabilize

Serves: 2

1 cup uncooked quinoa

½ teaspoon fine sea salt, plus more to taste

2 tablespoons lemon juice

1 garlic clove, minced

½ cup extra-virgin olive oil

⅛ teaspoon dried oregano

⅛ teaspoon dried coriander

Ground black pepper to taste

Red pepper flakes (optional)

½ (14-ounce) can of salmon (wild Alaskan, in water), drained

1 cucumber, chopped

1 pint cherry tomatoes, sliced in half

⅔ cup flat-leaf parsley, chopped

¼ cup fresh mint, chopped

1 scallion, finely chopped

1. Bring the quinoa, the ½ teaspoon salt, and 1¼ cups water to a boil in a medium saucepan over high heat. Reduce the heat to medium-low, cover, and simmer until the quinoa is tender, about 10 minutes.
2. Whisk the lemon juice and garlic in a small bowl. Whisk in the olive oil. Add the oregano and coriander, and season to taste with salt, black pepper, and red pepper flakes.
3. Add the salmon to the dressing to marinate quickly while you complete the preparation.
4. Combine the cucumber, tomatoes, parsley, mint, and scallion in a bowl. Add the quinoa and mix.
5. Pour the dressing and salmon over the quinoa and toss. Add salt and pepper as needed.

Notes:

- You can substitute leftover cooked salmon for canned.
- You can use precooked frozen quinoa that you heat on the stovetop or in the microwave.

36. PRESSURE COOKER LENTIL SOUP WITH SPINACH

(An Instant Pot or similar pressure cooker works great for this!)

Lentils are a legume that is loaded with protein and fiber, so they give you lots of sustained energy. And they taste amazing when prepared with onion, carrots, and celery. This is a simple soup that just never gets old.

Phase: Scrub, Soak Up, Stabilize
Serves: 4

2 teaspoons avocado oil

1 cup diced yellow onion

1 cup diced carrots

½ cup diced celery

3 garlic cloves, minced

2 teaspoons cumin

1 teaspoon coriander

1 teaspoon dried thyme

½ teaspoon salt

Black pepper to taste

1 cup dry brown lentils

4 cups vegetable broth (low-sodium)

5 cups baby spinach

1. Press the sauté button on the Instant Pot and add the oil. When hot, add the onion, carrots, and celery. Sauté, stirring occasionally, until tender, about 5 minutes. Add the garlic, cumin, coriander, thyme, salt, and pepper to taste. Cook, stirring constantly, for 1 to 2 minutes more.

2. Add the lentils and pour in the broth. Stir.

3. Place the lid on the Instant Pot and make sure the release valve is in the sealing position. Set the timer at 12 minutes and allow to cook.

4. When done, flip the quick-release valve to vent. Once venting is complete, remove the lid and stir in the spinach. Taste and add additional salt and pepper if desired. Serve immediately.

Notes:

If you don't have an Instant Pot but instead another multi-cooker or pressure cooker without a sauté function, you can do the sauté step on the stovetop, cooking until onions become translucent, then transfer the veggies to the pressure cooker. This soup keeps well refrigerated for 3 days.

37. COZY CREAMY CHICKEN STEW

I replaced heavy (dairy) cream with coconut milk and cashews in this classic stew recipe. If that doesn't sound appealing at first, just give it a try. You won't regret it.

Phase: Stabilize

Serves: 4

2 tablespoons olive oil

1 cup diced onion

1 cup diced carrots

1 cup diced celery

5 garlic cloves, minced

2 cups chicken broth (organic if possible)

1 cup cauliflower florets, chopped medium

1½ teaspoons dried sage

½ teaspoon dried thyme

2 large boneless, skinless chicken breasts, chopped into bite-size pieces

½ cup coconut milk

1 cup cashews

1 teaspoon fine sea salt or more to taste

Fresh cracked black pepper to taste

1. Heat the oil in a large saucepan over medium heat. Sauté the onion, carrots, and celery until the onion is soft and translucent. Add the garlic and sauté about a minute more.
2. Add the broth, cauliflower, sage, and thyme, and bring to a simmer.
3. Add the chicken and cook for about 6 minutes, until the chicken is cooked through.
4. Place the coconut milk and cashews in a blender. Blend on high until very smooth.
5. Pour the cashew-coconut cream into the pan with the chicken and stir well. Season with salt and pepper.

Notes:
- To reduce creaminess, blend the cashews with ½ cup water and leave out the coconut milk.
- Coconut milk and cashews can turn any soup into a cream-based soup without the use of dairy. This is a rich and delicious replacement for heavy cream.

I think the mason jar is one of the most underappreciated tools in the kitchen. It's such a great way to make and portion out meals ahead of time so you can grab and go later on. I love this recipe for all of its fiber and flavor.

Phase: Scrub, Soak Up, Stabilize
(depending on ingredients you choose)

Serves: 1

¼ cup beans of choice (canned or precooked) or quinoa (precooked)

2 tablespoons dressing of choice or salsa

½ cup chicken breast (cooked and diced)

¼ cup tomato, cucumber, bell pepper, carrots, beets, or celery, chopped/diced (choose one or a combination)

¼ cup romaine or spring mix

1. If using the precooked quinoa, heat on the stovetop or in the microwave.
2. In a pint-size mason jar, layer the ingredients in the order listed above until all five have been added.
3. When ready to eat, shake the jar and pour into a bowl. Enjoy!

Notes:

Try topping it with a few avocado slices or shredded low-fat/fat-free cheese. You can forgo the beans/quinoa and increase one or more of the other parts. Make a few of these lunches at a time for the following few days of the week.

39. ONE-PAN CHICKEN AND VEGGIES

The lemon slices and avocado oil really add dimension to this dish, which is easy to make and always a crowd pleaser.

Phase: Stabilize

Serves: 2

2 large chicken breasts

Sea salt and black pepper to taste

½ lemon, sliced into rounds

2 cups sliced carrots,

sliced semi-thick on the diagonal

3 cups broccoli

2 tablespoons avocado oil

1. Preheat the oven to 375°F and line a baking sheet with foil.
2. Place the chicken breasts in the middle of the baking sheet, sprinkle with salt and pepper, and top with the sliced lemon.
3. Mix the carrots and broccoli with the oil and add salt to taste.
4. Arrange the veggies around the chicken on the baking sheet.
5. Bake for 30 minutes, or until the chicken is cooked through.

Notes:

- If your carrots are very thick, cut them in half lengthwise before cutting them on the diagonal.
- Use a poultry thermometer to check for internal temperature. Remove the chicken from the oven once it reaches 165°F, to avoid overcooking and to maximize flavor and tenderness.

40. TURKEY BOLOGNESE OVER ZUCCHINI NOODLES

Yes, you really can enjoy a delicious Italian-style meal without blowing your diet. This Bolognese is rich and decadent, and I think you'll love how it tastes with zucchini noodles.

Phase: Stabilize

Serves: 4

1 tablespoon olive oil

1 pound ground lean turkey

¾ (24-ounce) jar (give or take a couple of ounces) of your favorite tomato/marinara/spaghetti sauce

1 (12-ounce) package refriger-ated zucchini noodles, or 4 whole zucchini

Cracked black pepper to taste

Grated part-skim Parmesan cheese to sprinkle on top (optional)

1. Heat the oil in a nonstick pan. Add the ground turkey, stirring to break it up as it cooks. After 5 minutes, add the tomato sauce. Cover and let simmer for about 10 minutes.
2. While the sauce is simmering, open the zucchini noodles and arrange on a plate. If using whole zucchini, spiralize them and arrange on the plate.
3. Pour the Bolognese sauce over the noodles. Top with pepper and/or Parmesan as desired.

Notes:

Most stores sell spiralized zucchini noodles, making this quick and simple recipe even faster. If you don't have that option or prefer to make your own, a countertop spiral slicer does the trick. If you prefer your zucchini noodles warmed, heat 1 tablespoon of olive oil in a large pan, add 1 teaspoon garlic and sauté for 30 seconds, then sauté the zucchini noodles for 5 minutes, until just tender.

41. TEMPEH SALAD

The sesame seed oil, soy sauce, and rice vinegar give this salad a distinctly Asian flavor, and I love the addition of radish for a little extra kick.

Phase: Soak Up, Stabilize

Serves: 1

4 ounces tempeh (half a standard package)

1 tablespoon soy sauce (low-sodium) or tamari

1 tablespoon rice vinegar

½ teaspoon sesame seed oil

2 teaspoons grated fresh ginger (optional)

½ garlic clove, minced

¼ cucumber, sliced

1 radish, sliced

3 tablespoons shredded carrots

2 cups mixed greens

2 teaspoons dressing of your choice with a sesame, miso, peanut, or vinaigrette base

1 teaspoon avocado oil

Sea salt and ground black pepper to taste

1. Chop the tempeh into bite-size cubes.
2. Combine the soy sauce, rice vinegar, sesame oil, ginger (if using), and garlic in a bowl and mix well to create a marinade.
3. Put the tempeh in the marinade and let sit at room temperature for 30 minutes.
4. Toss the cucumber, radish, carrots, and greens in a bowl, and add the dressing.
5. Heat the avocado oil in a pan over medium-high heat. Add the tempeh pieces and marinade and sauté until golden brown, about 5 minutes.
6. Top the salad with tempeh. Season with salt and pepper to taste.

42. TURKEY AND KALE SAUTÉ

This simple dish can be thrown together in just a few minutes, and you can personalize it with your favorite seasonings.

Phase: Soak Up, Stabilize

Serves: 2

1 teaspoon avocado oil

½ white onion, chopped

2 garlic cloves, minced

1 cup crimini mushrooms, chopped

8 ounces ground turkey

½ teaspoon dried oregano

½ teaspoon dried thyme

¼ cup vegetable broth

2 cups kale, chopped

Sea salt to taste

Cracked black pepper to taste

1. In a sauté pan, heat the avocado oil over medium heat. Add the onion, garlic, and mushrooms, and cook until the onion is translucent, about 4 minutes.
2. Add the ground turkey, oregano, and thyme, plus salt and pepper to taste. Continue to cook for about 5 minutes, breaking it up as it cooks.
3. Pour the vegetable broth over the turkey.
4. Add the kale and additional salt and pepper to taste. Cook until the kale is slightly wilted, approximately 5 minutes, and allow to simmer for a few more minutes, until the turkey cooks through.

Notes:

This is satisfying on its own, or serve it over quinoa, cauliflower rice, or zucchini noodles, or with squash or sweet potatoes. A squeeze of lemon brings out even more flavor!

43. ONE-PAN CHICKEN, BROCCOLINI, AND SQUASH

Broccolini is one of my favorite vegetables. I really love it in this recipe, which is reminiscent of a delicious French-style roasted chicken, thanks to the rosemary.

Phase: Soak Up, Stabilize

Serves: 2

1 (8-ounce) boneless, skinless chicken breast

2 cups chopped broccolini

2 cups chopped yellow squash

2 tablespoons extra-virgin olive oil

1 lemon, juiced

½ tablespoon rosemary

Sea salt to taste

Cracked black pepper to taste

1. Preheat the oven to 400°F and line a baking sheet with parchment paper. Place the chicken breast, broccolini, and squash on the baking sheet.
2. In a small bowl, mix together the oil, lemon juice, rosemary, salt, and pepper. Mix well, then drizzle over the chicken and vegetables.
3. Bake for 25 to 30 minutes, or until the chicken is cooked through.

Notes:

Use a poultry thermometer to check for doneness; when the chicken's internal temperature reaches 165°F, remove it from the oven to avoid overcooking.

44. CAULIFLOWER PIZZA NIGHT

Who doesn't love pizza night? Have a little fun with this and add any combination of toppings. You can make this a super-deluxe veggie pizza by piling on all your favorite vegetables. Or throw in some pineapple for a little sweetness!

Phase: Stabilize

Serves: 2

1 cauliflower pizza crust (store-bought)

½ cup pizza sauce

½ cup spinach or arugula

1 to 2 fresh basil leaves, chopped (optional)

6 to 8 cherry tomatoes, sliced in half

2 to 4 ounces grilled chicken (cooked and diced)

Shredded part-skim mozzarella to taste (optional)

Grated Parmesan to taste (optional)

½ teaspoon dried oregano

Red pepper flakes to taste (optional)

1. Follow the directions for baking the pizza crust, usually 400°F for 10 minutes.
2. Remove the crust from the oven and add the toppings. You can serve immediately, or put the pizza back in the oven for 2 minutes and then serve.

Notes:

Cauliflower has so many different uses, and pizza crust is one of the most popular. There are multiple brands that offer cauli pizza crusts, so take your pick.

45. TERIYAKI-GLAZED DRUMSTICKS

Often, teriyaki-style dishes have a lot of added sugar, so they aren't diet-friendly, but this recipe sidesteps the sugar with the addition of honey. All the flavor, none of the guilt!

Phase: Stabilize

Serves: 4

1½ cups soy sauce (low-sodium) or tamari sauce

2 tablespoons mirin vinegar

¼ cup honey

2 teaspoons sesame oil

1 tablespoon garlic, minced

½ tablespoon grated fresh ginger

1 teaspoon crushed red pepper flakes (optional)

2 pounds chicken drumsticks

1. In a large mixing bowl, combine all the ingredients except the chicken. Whisk well. Set aside ½ cup of the sauce.
2. Place the chicken in a large resealable plastic bag. Pour the marinade over the chicken, seal the bag, and adjust to ensure that the drumsticks are evenly coated. Marinate in the refrigerator for at least 1 hour, or overnight for more flavor.
3. Preheat the oven to 375°F.
4. Arrange the chicken on a baking sheet lined with parchment paper, making sure to empty all the sauce from the plastic bag over the drumsticks.
5. Bake uncovered for 45 to 50 minutes, until the chicken is cooked through. Add the remaining ½ cup sauce in the last 5 minutes of baking or right after you remove the dish from the oven.

Notes:

You can replace the honey with an equal amount of monk fruit sweetener. For a quicker recipe, replace the homemade sauce with 1½ cups of a low-carb store-bought teriyaki sauce (as low-carb as possible, with less than 5 grams of sugar per serving and preferably less than 3 grams). This recipe works great over cauliflower rice, or served with broccoli or mixed veggies.

46. SALMON KABOBS

When you're in the mood to fire up the grill, these kabobs are the perfect meal to make. The red pepper flakes give them just the right amount of heat, and the lemon complements the flavor of the salmon beautifully.

Phase: Scrub, Soak Up, Stabilize
Serves: 4

Avocado oil cooking spray as needed for the grill

1 tablespoon chopped fresh oregano

1 tablespoon chopped fresh parsley

2 teaspoons sesame seeds

1 teaspoon cumin

¼ teaspoon red pepper flakes

1 teaspoon fine sea salt

1¼ pounds salmon fillet (preferably wild), sliced into 1-inch cubes

2 lemons, thinly sliced into rounds

8 barbecue skewers

1. Heat the grill to medium-hot and spray the grates with cooking spray.
2. Combine the oregano, parsley, sesame seeds, cumin, red pepper flakes, and salt in a small bowl.
3. Dredge the salmon pieces in the spice mixture, covering evenly.
4. Slide a piece of salmon onto a skewer, followed by a folded lemon slice, and repeat. The recipe should provide enough salmon to fill eight skewers.
5. Grill the fish, turning occasionally, until the salmon is opaque throughout, 8 to 10 minutes.

Notes:

You can also add veggies like asparagus, bell peppers, and onions to the grill to eat with the kabobs.

News flash: chicken nuggets aren't just for kids! This grain-free, grown-up version of the childhood classic is a tasty way to get your protein for the day. Yum!

Phase: Soak Up, Stabilize

Serves: 4

1 pound chicken tenderloins	1 teaspoon onion powder
1 cup almond flour	¼ teaspoon black pepper
1 teaspoon fine sea salt	1 egg
1 teaspoon smoked paprika	3 tablespoons avocado oil
½ teaspoon garlic powder	

1. Cut the chicken tenderloins into 1- to 2-inch bite-size pieces.
2. In a small mixing bowl, combine the almond flour, salt, paprika, garlic powder, onion powder, and pepper, and mix well.
3. In a separate bowl, crack the egg and whisk with a fork.
4. Heat a large frying pan or cast-iron skillet over medium heat and add the oil.
5. Dip each chicken piece into the egg, moistening well, and then into the almond flour mixture, coating on all sides. Divide the pieces into two batches.
6. Cook the first batch of chicken in the frying pan, 2 to 4 minutes on each side or until just cooked through, adjusting the heat to avoid burning the outside. Cook the second batch, adding more oil as needed.
7. Transfer the nuggets to a paper towel–covered plate to absorb any excess oil.

Notes:
- If your egg is small, use a second egg.
- These nuggets work great on top of a large mixed green or romaine salad with cucumbers and tomatoes, or serve with a cup or two of your favorite veggies. Delicious!

This shrimp stew will make you look like a gourmet chef even though it's incredibly easy to make.

Phase: Soak Up, Stabilize

Serves: 3

1 cup shrimp, peeled and deveined

½ teaspoon fine sea salt

1 tablespoon extra-virgin olive oil

½ red or green bell pepper, sliced into thin strips

2 scallions (bulbs only), sliced

⅓ cup cilantro, chopped

2 garlic cloves, coarsely chopped

¼ teaspoon red pepper flakes

½ (14-ounce) can diced tomatoes (drained)

½ (13.5-ounce) can light coconut milk

1 tablespoon lime juice

1. In a bowl, sprinkle the shrimp with salt and toss to coat evenly. Set aside.
2. Heat the oil in a large nonstick pot over medium heat. Add the bell pepper and cook, stirring, until almost tender, about 4 minutes.
3. Add the scallions, cilantro, garlic, and red pepper flakes. Continue to cook, stirring, for another minute.
4. Add the tomatoes and coconut milk and bring to a simmer. Reduce the heat to medium and simmer for 5 minutes.
5. Add the shrimp and continue to cook, partially covered and stirring frequently, until they are cooked through, about 5 minutes. Add the lime juice and season to taste with salt. You can also garnish with any additional cilantro or the chopped leftover scallion greens.

Notes:

This hearty stew can be eaten on its own or with/over additional cooked veggies, cauliflower rice, or quinoa. Or add a salad on the side.

If you love tacos with ground beef, I think you'll be surprised how well turkey works as a substitute! All of these flavors come together really well, and I love using lettuce cups instead of taco shells. I think you will too!

Phase: Stabilize

Serves: 4

1 tablespoon avocado oil

½ yellow onion, diced

1 pound lean ground turkey

1 ounce taco seasoning (your favorite)

1 tablespoon lime juice

10 cherry tomatos, sliced in half

1 jalapeño, seeds removed and chopped

1 head iceberg or romaine lettuce (leaves pulled apart and washed)

1 avocado, cubed

1. In a large pan, heat the oil over medium-high heat. Add the onion and cook for about 5 minutes, until translucent.
2. Add the ground turkey, breaking it into very small pieces, and cook until no longer pink.
3. Add the taco seasoning and lime juice and stir until the turkey is coated evenly.
4. Add half the tomatoes and all of the jalapeño. Stir to combine, and cook for another 5 minutes, until the tomatoes are soft. Remove from the heat.
5. Divide the turkey among the lettuce leaves, and top with the remaining tomatoes and the avocado.

Notes:

Garnish with cilantro, extra jalapeños, and any other of your favorite toppings.

Poaching is a great cooking method for chicken, leaving it extra tender and juicy. The addition of sake or sherry and some ginger really puts it over the top!

Phase: Stabilize

Serves: 1

4 to 6 ounces boneless, skinless chicken breast

Filtered water to cover chicken for poaching

2 teaspoons fine sea salt

Splash of sherry or sake

1-inch piece fresh ginger (sliced with skin)

1. Use a medium pan that is deep enough to hold the chicken breast plus enough water to barely cover.
2. Put the water, salt, a splash of sherry, and the piece of ginger into the pan.
3. Add the chicken breast and turn on the heat. Bring to a boil, then turn over the chicken. Turn off the heat and pull the pan completely off the heat.
4. Cover the pan with a tight-fitting lid and let it rest for about 10 minutes, depending on how big the chicken breast is.
5. Poke the center of the chicken; it should be bouncy and slightly yielding, not rock-hard. If it feels too soft, poke a hole and peek inside. If it's a bit too pink, put the lid back on and leave for another 5 to 10 minutes. (A poultry thermometer can help you check for doneness and avoid overcooking; look for an internal temperature of 165°F.)

Notes:

Combine with 1 to 2 cups of vegetables of your choice. Double the recipe for 2 servings.

51. CURRIED BROILED FISH

Looking for a quick dinner that doesn't involve the microwave? You can have a delicious, satisfying meal in just 15 minutes with this recipe. So easy. So good. So, go for it!

Phase: Scrub, Soak Up, Stabilize

Serves: 1

4 to 6 ounces whitefish

½ lemon

1 teaspoon curry seasoning

1 slice of tomato

1. Preheat the broiler for 10 minutes.
2. Squeeze the juice from the lemon over the fish, sprinkle with curry seasoning, and top with the tomato slice.
3. Place the fish on the broiler rack 8 to 10 inches away from heat source. Broil for 10 to 15 minutes, or until the tomato starts to blacken. Serve while hot.

Notes:

Leftovers can be refrigerated for up to 2 days, but no longer. Simply double the recipe for 2 servings.

The bright flavors of orange, honey, and lemon make this salad a star. Especially if you eat a lot of chicken and you're looking to change it up, turkey is a fantastic alternative. Enjoy!

Phase: Stabilize

Serves: 4 to 6

2 oranges with peels on, sliced medium-thick

1 white onion, quartered

3 pounds turkey breast (skin-on and bone in, fresh or completely thawed)

2 teaspoons fine sea salt

2½ tablespoons olive oil

1 tablespoon chopped fresh thyme

1 tablespoon chopped fresh sage

½ tablespoon chopped fresh rosemary

1 cup filtered water

For the dressing

¼ cup extra-virgin olive oil

Juice of ½ orange

Juice of ½ lemon

1½ teaspoons honey

Pinch of orange zest

Mixed greens (2 cups per serving)

1. Place a rack in the bottom third of the oven and heat oven to 450°F.
2. Arrange the orange slices and onion quarters in a large baking dish or roasting pan.
3. Season the turkey breast on all sides with the salt, then place it on top of the orange slices and onion in the pan.
4. Combine the 2½ tablespoons olive oil with the thyme, sage, and rosemary in a small mixing bowl. Pour over the turkey breast.
5. Add the water to the bottom of the pan. Lower the oven temperature to 350°F and bake the turkey for 60 minutes. At about 40 minutes, begin checking the turkey for an internal temperature of 165°F. The skin should be brown and crispy. Add more water to the pan if it evaporates too quickly or if the pan starts to burn.

6. Once the turkey is done, let cool for 15 minutes before slicing.
7. For the citrus dressing, whisk together the ¼ cup extra-virgin olive oil, orange juice, lemon juice, honey, and pinch of zest until blended well. This should be enough for 3 to 6 salads. The dressing will keep in the refrigerator for up to 1 week, preferably stored in a mason jar.
8. For each serving, slice 4 to 6 ounces of turkey breast, place over 2 cups mixed greens, and add 2 tablespoons or more of citrus dressing.

Notes:

You can substitute monk fruit for honey in the dressing recipe if preferred.

53. QUICK BAKED SOLE

Sole is a light, subtle-tasting fish, and in this recipe, the paprika really brings it to life. And preparing it in the oven makes it so simple.

Phase: Scrub, Soak Up, Stabilize

Serves: 4

½ teaspoon garlic salt

½ teaspoon paprika

3 tablespoons extra-virgin olive oil

1 pound sole fillets

½ lemon

Fine sea salt and black pepper to taste

1. Preheat the oven to 375°F.
2. Mix the garlic salt, paprika, and oil in a bowl.
3. Place the sole fillets in a baking dish and pour the oil mixture over them.
4. Squeeze the juice from the lemon half over the fillets and season with salt and pepper.
5. Bake for 20 minutes, until flaky.

Notes:

Combine with 1 to 2 cups of any favorite in-season vegetables or a side salad.

54. CAULIFLOWER FRIED RICE

Using one of my favorite multipurpose ingredients, cauliflower, this twist on fried rice is sure to surprise and delight any crowd.

Phase: Soak Up, Stabilize

Serves: 4

2 tablespoons toasted sesame oil

2 garlic cloves, minced

1 tablespoon minced fresh ginger

1 carrot, diced

1 cup frozen peas

4 eggs

1 (10-ounce) bag frozen cauliflower rice

1 tablespoon honey

3 tablespoons low-sodium soy sauce or tamari sauce

¼ cup cashews, chopped (optional)

2 green onions, chopped

1. Heat a large nonstick skillet on medium-high. Add the oil and coat evenly. Then add the garlic, ginger, carrot, and peas and cook for 4 to 5 minutes, stirring occasionally.
2. Push the vegetables to one side and add the eggs to the other side of the same skillet. Cook until scrambled.
3. Add the cauliflower rice to the skillet, stir, and cook until warmed through.
4. Add the honey, soy sauce, and cashews, if using. Mix the entire dish together in the skillet for an additional 1 to 2 minutes.
5. Sprinkle with green onions.

Notes:
- This meal is complete; the eggs serve as the protein. However, if you want to add an additional protein or leave out the eggs, you can use 4 to 6 ounces of chopped chicken breast for chicken fried rice or the same amount of shrimp for shrimp fried rice.
- Add the cauliflower rice direct from the freezer. If it thaws ahead, the rice could get soggy.
- You can replace the honey with maple syrup or liquid monk fruit.

WATER INFUSION RECIPES

Since hydration is so key for this program and for good health in general, I wanted to spark some ideas in case you're one of those people who can't stand to drink plain water. Now you'll have no excuse! These are smart ways to infuse your water with flavor, without adding sugar or sweetener. For all of these water infusions, fill a jug or pitcher with 8 cups of filtered water, then add the listed ingredients. The longer they remain in the water, the more potent the flavors become. You can remove the ingredients if it's getting too strong. Alternatively, you can purchase a water-infusing pitcher or bottle. There are lots of options available these days. Carry it around with you wherever you go so that you stay perfectly hydrated throughout your day. Drink up!

(And remember, if you often wake up at night to go pee, stop drinking fluids at least a couple hours before bedtime.)

Ginger Citrus Water

Fresh gingerroot, peeled and chopped into large chunks

1 lemon, sliced thinly

Place the ginger and lemon slices in a pitcher and fill with 8 cups water. Keep in the refrigerator for up to 2 days. Enjoy!

Cinnamon Apple Water

2 cinnamon sticks

1 green apple, cored and sliced into circles

1. You can drop the cinnamon sticks right into the pitcher, or simmer them on the stove for 5 minutes first to really unlock the flavor.
2. Place the cinnamon sticks and apple slices in a pitcher and fill with 8 cups water. Keep in the refrigerator for up to 2 days. Enjoy!

Spicy Water

Fresh cilantro, chopped

½ fresh jalapeño, sliced
and seeds removed (or

keep the seeds for mega
spice)

1 lime, sliced thinly

Place the cilantro, jalapeño, and lime slices in a pitcher and fill with 8 cups of water. Keep in the refrigerator for up to 2 days. Enjoy!

Strawberry Kiwi Mint Water

8 to 10 strawberries,
cut in half

2 kiwis, peeled

and cut into circles

1 handful fresh
mint

Place the strawberries, kiwis, and mint in a pitcher and fill with 8 cups water. Keep in the refrigerator for up to 2 days. Enjoy!

Vanilla Lemongrass Water

8 drops pure vanilla extract (not
imitation)

1 or 2 sprigs fresh lemongrass

Place the lemongrass in a pitcher and fill with 8 cups water. Add the vanilla. Keep in the refrigerator for up to 2 days. Enjoy!

Rosemary Lavender Water

2 sprigs fresh rosemary

2 sprigs fresh lavender

Place the rosemary and lavender in a pitcher and fill with 8 cups water. Keep in the refrigerator for up to 2 days. Enjoy!

Mixed Berry Water

1 handful blackberries

1 handful raspberries

1 handful blueberries

Muddle the berries in the bottom of a pitcher with a spoon to bring out the flavors. Fill with 8 cups water. Keep in the refrigerator for up to 2 days. Enjoy!

Piña Colada Water

1 cup chopped pineapple   1 cup coconut chunks

Place the pineapple and coconut in a pitcher and fill with 8 cups filtered water. Keep in the refrigerator for up to 2 days. Enjoy!

Citrus Water

1 orange, thinly sliced   1 lime, thinly sliced
1 lemon, thinly sliced

Place all the citrus slices in a pitcher and fill with 8 cups filtered water. Keep in the refrigerator for up to 2 days. Enjoy!

Cucumber Water

1 cucumber, thinly sliced   2 sprigs fresh mint

Place the cucumber slices and mint in a pitcher and fill with 8 cups filtered water. Keep in the refrigerator for up to 2 days. Enjoy!

17 DAYS OF SAMPLE MENUS

3 Days of Scrub

*Don't forget to stay hydrated and get your 64 to 100 ounces of water a day!

Day 1

Breakfast: Green Omega Smoothie

Snack (midmorning or midafternoon): ½ cup hummus with cucumbers and celery OR 1 cup bone broth

Lunch: Avocado Smoked Salmon Wrap

Beverage: Nettle leaf tea

Dinner: Pressure Cooker Lentil Soup with Spinach

Day 2

Breakfast: 1 tablespoon sunflower butter mixed with 2 teaspoons honey, with ½ cup blueberries mixed in

Snack (midmorning or midafternoon): 1 cup coconut water OR Banana Berry "Ice Cream"

Lunch: Homemade hummus (chickpeas, turmeric, paprika, olive oil) + cucumber and zucchini "chips" + three-bean salad (mix three different types of beans with 2 teaspoons olive oil)

Beverage: Dandelion coffee

Dinner: Curried Broiled Fish, avocado/cilantro salad atop arugula with lemon juice

Day 3

Breakfast: Overnight Chia Pudding

Snack (midmorning or midafternoon): Berry cup (your choice of blueberries, raspberries, strawberries, or blackberries, topped with a dash of cinnamon) OR Kale Crunchies

Lunch: Avocado Crunch Tartines, Quick Celery and Parsley Detox Salad

Beverage: 8 ounces fresh vegetable juice (cucumber, celery, ginger, lemon)

Dinner: Easy Creamy Tomato Soup, In a Snap Pea Salad and 5-Minute Dressing

4 Days of Soak Up

Day 4

Breakfast: 1 slice Soak It Up Seed Bread, 1 medium boiled egg, pinch of sea salt and black pepper

Snack (midmorning or midafternoon): Banana slices with 1 tablespoon sunflower butter OR Matcha Ginger Latte with coconut or hemp milk

Lunch: Quinoa, green pea, and mixed veggie "stir-fry"

Beverage: Citrus Water

Dinner: Veggie chili with beans, zucchini, bell peppers, chili powder, diced sweet potato

Day 5

Breakfast: Smoothie made with coconut milk, frozen blueberries, cinnamon, hemp or chia seeds, 2 teaspoons honey

Snack (midmorning or midafternoon): ABC Pudding OR Lemon-Cucumber-Mint Detox Aid

Lunch: Quick Salmon Salad, flaxseed crackers

Beverage: Rosemary Lavender Water

Dinner: Egg Muffins, My Big Italian Veggie Bake

Day 6

Breakfast: Cooked hot quinoa porridge with coconut milk and berries
Snack (midmorning or midafternoon): Cherry Soak Pops OR 8 ounces fresh vegetable juice (cucumber, celery, ginger, lemon)
Lunch: Black Bean Salad in lettuce cups, topped with salsa
Beverage: Ginger Citrus Water
Dinner: Chipotle Fish Tacos

Day 7

Breakfast: Green Omega Smoothie
Snack (midmorning or midafternoon): ½ cup frozen grapes OR 1 cup diced jicama (add a dash of lemon or lime juice)
Lunch: Quinoa Tabouli with Salmon
Beverage: Cinnamon Apple Water
Dinner: Garlicky Tuscan Beans and Swiss Greens

10 Days of Stabilize

Day 8

Breakfast: 1 cup slow-cooked steel cut oatmeal topped with 6 walnuts and a drizzle of honey or maple syrup
Snack (midmorning or midafternoon): Red grapes OR a boiled egg and cut-up veggies
Lunch: Protein-Powered Veggie Soup
Beverage: Mixed Berry Water
Dinner: Turkey Bolognese over Zucchini Noodles

Day 9

Breakfast: Egg Muffins
Snack (midmorning or midafternoon): Mandarin slices OR 12 roasted almonds
Lunch: Quick Mason Jar Lunch in 5 Parts
Beverage: Coconut water
Dinner: Turkey and Kale Sauté, Roasted Acorn Squash and Shallots

Day 10

Breakfast: Sweet Potato Toast

Snack (midmorning or midafternoon): ½ cup berries OR carrots and celery with ½ cup cashew cheese dip

Lunch: Poached Chicken Breast with Veggies

Beverage: Vanilla Lemongrass Water

Dinner: Cauliflower Pizza Night

Day 11

Breakfast: 1 slice of sprouted bread, 1 tablespoon almond butter, 1 teaspoon apple butter, 1 poached egg

Snack (midmorning or midafternoon): 1 small orange OR 12 cashews

Lunch: Baked Mustard Chicken, Rainbow Sesame Coleslaw

Beverage: Strawberry Kiwi Mint Water

Dinner: Salmon Kabobs

Day 12

Breakfast: Yogurt (organic dairy or plant-based) with ½ cup berries

Snack (midmorning or midafternoon): 1 serving dried plums or prunes OR 1 single-serving bag of crunchy chickpeas or lupini snacking beans

Lunch: Sardines mashed with dill relish, drizzled with olive oil, and seasoned to taste, with seed crackers or 1 slice sourdough bread

Beverage: Herbal chai tea with a splash of unsweetened cashew milk

Dinner: One-Pan Chicken and Veggies

Day 13

Breakfast: 1 whole egg and 1 egg white scrambled with 1 cup Easy Greens Sauté

Snack (midmorning or midafternoon): 1 serving prunes OR no-bake protein balls (oats, peanut butter, and honey)

Lunch: Tempeh Salad

Beverage: Piña Colada Water

Dinner: Teriyaki-Glazed Drumsticks, Cauliflower Fried Rice

Day 14

Breakfast: Green Omega Smoothie

Snack (midmorning or midafternoon): 1 pear OR 6 pecans

Lunch: Steak Salad with No-Oil Lemon Dressing

Beverage: Green tea

Dinner: One-Pot Shrimp Stew

Day 15

Breakfast: Almond Flour Pancakes

Snack (midmorning or midafternoon): Green apple and 1 tablespoon almond butter OR thin-sliced raw carrots and beets

Lunch: Chickpea Salad, served with seed crackers or whole rye crispbread

Beverage: Kombucha

Dinner: One-Pan Chicken, Broccolini, and Squash, 1 tablespoon sauerkraut

Day 16

Breakfast: High-Protein Porridge

Snack (midmorning or midafternoon): 1 peach OR 8 ounces fresh vegetable juice (cucumber, celery, ginger, lemon)

Lunch: Loaded Turkey Tacos in Lettuce Cups, Simple Avocado Salad

Beverage: Citrus Water

Dinner: Cozy Creamy Chicken Stew

Day 17

Breakfast: Overnight Chia Pudding with berries and 1 tablespoon almond butter

Snack (midmorning or midafternoon): 1 plum OR a few cubes of organic grass-fed cheddar cheese and a couple of pickle slices

Lunch: White Bean and Tempeh Curry

Beverage: Spicy Water

Dinner: Crispy Healthy Chicken Nuggets, Baked Sweet Potato Fries, simple mixed-greens salad

ACKNOWLEDGMENTS

Words cannot describe my sense of gratitude to my dear friend Lisa Clark. Without her endless hours of dedication to this project, this guide to a better body would not exist. Her passion for health and wellness and, most of all, her kind and brilliant soul were essential to the completion of this project.

I would also like to thank Leona West Fox, the extremely talented nutritionist who helped shape the food plans and recipes in this book. She took the strong foundation of *The 17 Day Diet* and built on it to create a delicious, practical, clean, and wonderfully nutritious eating plan.

I am also deeply grateful to my dear friend Felicia Pagesh for all of her contributions to this project behind the scenes. She keeps me in line!

And to Leah Miller and the incredible team at Simon & Schuster, you believed in this concept from day one, and I know how lucky I am to have the best publisher in the game behind me. You are a top-notch team, but over and above that, you are gifted collaborators. I always feel encouraged and supported by you, and that is priceless.

And of course, thank you, Shannon Marven and Rebecca Silensky of Dupree Miller, the world-class literary agency. Shannon, you are a creative force unlike any I've ever seen in action, and your ability to bring people together to make ideas come to life is without compare. Thank you for your tireless efforts on my behalf over many years of working together.

Saving the best for last, I'd like to send out a sincere thanks to all of my patients and my social media community for allowing me to be part of their lives. Together, we will make this world a healthier, happier place.

NOTES

CHAPTER 1: THE KICKSTART PHILOSOPHY

1 E. Battaglia Richi, B. Baumer, B. Conrad, R. Darioli, A. Schmid, and U. Keller, "Health Risks Associated with Meat Consumption: A Review of Epidemiological Studies," *International Journal for Vitamin and Nutrition Research* 85, no. 1/2 (2015): 70–8, https://doi.org/10.1024/0300-9831/a000224, PMID: 26780279.

2 US Department of Health and Human Services and US Department of Agriculture, *2015–2020 Dietary Guidelines for Americans*, 8th ed. (2017), https://doi.org/10.1097/nhh.0000000000000520.

CHAPTER 3: THE 3-DAY "SCRUB"

1 S. Sreelatha and R. Inbavalli, "Antioxidant, Antihyperglycemic, and Antihyperlipidemic Effects of *Coriandrum sativum* Leaf and Stem in Alloxan-Induced Diabetic Rats," *Journal of Food Science* 77, no. 7 (July 2012): T119–23, https://doi.org/10.1111/j.1750-3841.2012.02755.x, Epub June 1, 2012, PMID: 22671941.

2 Y. Omura and S. L. Beckman, "Role of Mercury (Hg) in Resistant Infections and Effective Treatment of *Chlamydia trachomatis* and *Herpes* Family Viral Infections (and Potential Treatment for Cancer) by Removing Localized Hg Deposits with Chinese Parsley and Delivering Effective Antibiotics Using Various Drug Uptake Enhancement Methods," *Acupuncture and Electro-Therapeutics Research* 20,

no. 3/4 (August/December 1995): 195–229, https://doi.org/10.3727 /036012995816357014, PMID: 8686573.

3 Stephanie Welton et al., "Intermittent Fasting and Weight Loss: Systematic Review," *Canadian Family Physician/Medecin de famille canadien* 66, no. 2 (2020): 117–25, PMID: 32060194.

CHAPTER 4: THE 4-DAY "SOAK UP"

1 L. O. Lee, P. James, and E. S. Zevon et al., "Optimism Is Associated with Exceptional Longevity in 2 Epidemiologic Cohorts of Men and Women," *Proceedings of the National Academy of Sciences of the USA* 116, no. 37 (2019): 18357–62, https://doi.org/10.1073 /pnas.1900712116.

CHAPTER 6: LET'S GET MOVING

1 E. Volpi, R. Nazemi, and S. Fujita, "Muscle Tissue Changes with Aging," *Current Opinion in Clinical Nutrition and Metabolic Care* 7, no. 4 (2004): 405–10, https://doi.org/10.1097/01.mco.0000134362.76653.b2.

2 S. Y. Yang, C. L. Shan, H. Qing, W. Wang, Y. Zhu, M. M. Yin, S. Machado, T. F. Yuan, and T. Wu, "The Effects of Aerobic Exercise on Cognitive Function of Alzheimer's Disease Patients," *CNS and Neurological Disorders–Drug Targets* 14, no. 10 (2015): 1292–7, https://doi.org /10.2174/1871527315666151111123319, PMID: 26556080.

3 R. Hashida, T. Kawaguchi, M. Bekki, M. Omoto, H. Matsuse, T. Nago, Y. Takano, T. Ueno, H. Koga, J. George, N. Shiba, and T. Torimura, "Aerobic vs. Resistance Exercise in Non-Alcoholic Fatty Liver Disease: A Systematic Review," *Journal of Hepatology* 66, no. 1 (January 2017): 142–52, https://doi.org/10.1016/j.jhep.2016.08.023, Epub September 14, 2016, PMID: 27639843.

CHAPTER 7: TO SUPPLEMENT OR NOT TO SUPPLEMENT?

1 Natural Marketing Institute, *2021 Supplements/OTC/Rx Consumer Trends and Insights Report*, 9th ed. (2020), accessed February 15, 2021, https://nmisolutions.com/research-reports/supplement-otc-rx-reports /usa/9th-edition-2021-supplements-otc-rx-consumer-trends-insights-report/.

2 Grand View Research, *Dietary Supplements Market Size, Share, and Trends Analysis Report by Ingredient (Vitamins, Minerals), by Form, by*

Application, by End User, by Distribution Channel, by Region, and Segment Forecasts, 2020–2027 (2020), accessed February 15, 2021, https://www.grandviewresearch.com/industry-analysis/dietary-supplements-market.

3 J. Mlcek, T. Jurikova, S. Skrovankova, and J. Sochor, "Quercetin and Its Anti-Allergic Immune Response," *Molecules* 21, no. 5 (May 12, 2016): 623, https://doi.org/10.3390/molecules21050623, PMID: 27187333, PMCID: PMC6273625.

4 National Center for Complementary and Integrative Health, "Melatonin: What You Need to Know," 2021, accessed February 15, 2021, https://www.nccih.nih.gov/health/melatonin-what-you-need-to-know.

CHAPTER 8: SLEEP YOURSELF SKINNY

1 Arlet V. Nedeltcheva et al., "Insufficient Sleep Undermines Dietary Efforts to Reduce Adiposity," *Annals of Internal Medicine* 153, no. 7 (2010): 435–41, https://doi.org/10.7326/0003-4819-153-7-201010050-00006.

2 V. Bayon, D. Leger, D. Gomez-Merino, M. F. Vecchierini, and M. Chennaoui, "Sleep Debt and Obesity," *Annals of Medicine* 46, no. 5 (August 2014): 264–72, https://doi.org/10.3109/07853890.2014.931103, Epub July 11, 2014, PMID: 25012962.

3 Michael A. Grandner et al., "Sleep Duration and Diabetes Risk: Population Trends and Potential Mechanisms," *Current Diabetes Reports* 16, no. 11 (2016): 106, https://doi.org/10.1007/s11892-016-0805-8.

4 National Institutes of Health, "How Disrupted Sleep May Lead to Heart Disease" (2019), accessed February 15, 2021, https://www.nih.gov/news-events/nih-research-matters/how-disrupted-sleep-may-lead-heart-disease.

5 K. Truong and D. Pacheco, "How Electronics Affect Sleep," Sleepfoundation.org, published November 6, 2020, accessed February 15, 2021, https://www.sleepfoundation.org/how-sleep-works/how-electronics-affect-sleep.

CHAPTER 9: BUILDING YOUR BENCH

1 L. C. Hawkley, R. A. Thisted, and J. T. Cacioppo, "Loneliness Predicts Reduced Physical Activity: Cross-Sectional and Longitudinal Analy-

ses," *Health Psychology* 28, no. 3 (2009): 354–63, https://doi.org/10.1037
/a0014400.

2 V. J. Felitti, R. F. Anda, D. Nordenberg, D. F. Williamson, A. M. Spitz, V. Edwards, M. P. Koss, and J. S. Marks, "Relationship of Childhood Abuse and Household Dysfunction to Many of the Leading Causes of Death in Adults: The Adverse Childhood Experiences (ACE) Study," *American Journal of Preventive Medicine* 14, no. 4 (May 1998): 245–58, https://doi.org/10.1016/s0749-3797(98)00017-8, PMID: 9635069.

3 B. R. Stork, N. J. Akselberg, Y. Qin, and D. C. Miller, "Adverse Childhood Experiences (ACEs) and Community Physicians: What We've Learned," *Permanente Journal* (2020) 24: 19.099, https://doi.org/10.7812 /TPP/19.099.

CHAPTER 10: WINNING YOUR BATTLE WITH STRESS

1 D. S. Krantz, B. Thorn, and J. Kiecolt-Glaser, "How Stress Affects Your Health," American Psychological Association, published 2013, accessed February 15, 2021, https://www.apa.org/topics/stress/health.

CHAPTER 11: THE CBD REVOLUTION

1 C. A. Sallaberry and L. Astern, "The Endocannabinoid System, Our Universal Regulator," *Journal of Young Investigators*, published June 1, 2018, accessed December 3, 2020, https://www.jyi.org/2018-june/2018 /6/1/the-endocannabinoid-system-our-universal-regulator.

2 Project CBD, "The Endocannabinoid System," accessed December 3, 2020, https://www.projectcbd.org/science/endocannabinoid-system.

3 "CBD: For Sleep and Insomnia," American Sleep Association, published 2019, accessed December 3, 2020, https://www.sleepassociation .org/sleep-treatments/cbd/.

4 P. G. Fine and M. J. Rosenfeld, "The Endocannabinoid System, Cannabinoids, and Pain," *Rambam Maimonides Medical Journal* 4, no. 4 (2013), https://doi.org/10.5041/rmmj.10129.

5 J. Johnson, "CBD for Weight Loss: Does It Work?" *Medical News Today*, published October 23, 2020, accessed December 3, 2020, https://www .medicalnewstoday.com/articles/324733#research.

6 S. Shannon, N. Lewis, H. Lee, and S. Hughes, "Cannabidiol in Anxiety and Sleep: A Large Case Series," *Permanente Journal* (2019) 23: 18–41, https://doi.org/10.7812/TPP/18-041.

7 N. Bruni, C. Della Pepa, S. Oliaro-Bosso, E. Pessione, D. Gastaldi, and F. Dosio, "Cannabinoid Delivery Systems for Pain and Inflammation Treatment," *Molecules* 23, no. 10 (2018): 2478, https://doi.org/10.3390/molecules23102478.

8 "Dietary Supplements and Herbal Medicines," United States Pharmacopeia, accessed February 15, 2021, https://www.usp.org/dietary-supplements-herbal-medicines.

INDEX

food list: last 10 days ("Stabilize"),
  66–72
foods to avoid, 30–36,
  67–68
fried foods, 67
fruits, 28, 36, 55, 57, 58, 68
"good" oils, 28, 35, 55, 69
guilty pleasures, 59
journaling, 58–61
juices, 76–77
oils, 28, 32, 35, 55, 69
for phase 1: 3-Day "Scrub,"
  25–47, 231–232
for phase 2: 4-Day "Soak-Up,"
  54–57, 232–233
for phase 3: 10-Day "Stabilize,"
  66–73, 233–235
Rule of 2's, 36, 37–40, 58
salt on, 41–42
sensitivity and intolerance,
  38
sleep and, 106, 110
spices, 29, 30, 40–41, 46, 56,
  57, 69
standard American diet (SAD), 3
vegetables, 27, 32, 45, 54, 57
"white" foods, 35, 67
whole grains, 68
See also beverages; meals;
  meat
Formula One: Drive to Survive
  (documentary), 20
4-Day "Soak Up" (phase 2),
  51–64
about, 51, 75
daily rhythm, 58
exercise, 52–53
food list for, 54–57
hunger, 52, 57
journaling, 58–61
Rule of 2's, 58
sample menus, 232–233
snacks, 52, 57, 58

starting the day, 58
tracking food choices,
  58–61
fried foods, 67
fries, recipe, 180
fruits
  adding to water, 76
  as dessert, 75
  food list, 28, 55, 58, 68
  juices, 76–77
  quercetin, 100–101
  Rule of 2's, 36, 37–40, 58
  as snack, 57
  when to eat, 36

G
garlic, 40
Garlicky Tuscan Beans and Swiss
  Greens (recipes), 172
ginger, 45
Ginger Citrus Water (recipe),
  227
glutes, exercises for, 94–95
goal setting, 155–163
grain-based foods
  eliminating, 26, 32, 35, 67
  whole grains, 68
Greek yogurt, 69
Green Omega Smoothie (recipe),
  169
green tea, 47, 56, 69, 76
grocery shopping, 72
guilt, 142
gut microbiome, 101

H
health
  childhood trauma and,
  124–125
  five pillars to good health, 7,
  108
  self-inventory, 158–161
  sleep and, 105

health status, self-inventory, 16–19
heel-toe walk, 90
high-glycemic foods, eliminating, 30, 32
High-Protein Porridge (recipe), 194
hip hinges (stretching exercise), 91
hunger
  4-Day "Soak Up," 52, 57
  3-Day "Scrub," 48–49
  tracking, 49
hydration. *See* beverages; drinking water
hydrogenated oils, 35

I

IBS (irritable bowel syndrome), 38
immunity, exercise and, 5
In A Snap Pea Salad and 5-Minute Dressing (recipe), 176
inflammation
  acute inflammation, 33–34
  chronic inflammation, 34
  foods causing, 26, 30, 32, 33–36
Instant Pot recipes, 206–207
intermittent fasting, 47–48
irritable bowel syndrome (IBS), 38

J
journaling, 58–61

K
Kale Crunchies (recipes), 185
kefir, 69, 101
kimchi, 101
knees, weight loss and, 15
kombucha, 76, 101

L
lactose intolerance, 38
laptops, sleep and, 106, 110
latte, recipe, 192
leafy greens
  17 Day Kickstart Diet, 27, 54, 68, 74
  recipes, 170–172, 185, 212
legs, exercises for, 94–95
legumes
  food list: first 3 days, 28, 55
  recipes, 176, 206–207
Lemon-Cucumber-Mint Detox Aid (recipe), 187
lemons, 41
liver, fatty liver, 7, 20–21, 82
Loaded Turkey Tacos in Lettuce Cups (recipe), 220
lunch
  bringing lunch to work, 72
  for 4-Day "Soak Up," 58
  recipes, 209
  sample menus, 231–235
  for 3-Day "Scrub," 36, 38–39
lunges, 94

M
M&M practice, 42, 44–45, 77–78
marijuana, 146
  See also CBD
Matcha Ginger Latte (recipe), 192
meal delivery services, 73
meals
  appetite, 149–150
  ideas for 3-Day "Scrub," 38–39
  planning, 72–73
  portion size, 40, 75
  sample menus, 231–235
  See also breakfast; dinner; lunch; recipes
meat
  about, 70–71
  allowable, 30–32, 69

chicken, 31, 57, 69, 199, 208, 210, 214, 218, 221
place in diet, 2
recipes, 191, 199, 208, 210, 211, 213, 214, 216
turkey, 211, 213, 220, 223–224
meditation, for stress management, 135–137
melatonin, 100
mental acuity, exercise and, 5, 82, 94
methylated B vitamins, 99
milk substitutes, food list:
first 3 days, 27, 54–55
mindfulness, 42, 44, 45, 77–78, 141–142
minerals. *See* nutritional supplements
mint, 41
Mixed Berry Water (recipe), 228
mocktails, 76
monk fruit, 29, 33
mood
CBD (cannabidiol) and, 146, 148, 150
exercise and, 5
motivation, 42, 44–45, 77–78, 88, 141–142
movement
benefits of, 5, 53, 81–83
brain and, 94
daily "Scrub" rhythm, 36
daily "Soak Up" rhythm, 58
motivation and, 44–45
routine for, 83–84
See also exercise
muscle mass, 81–82
music, for exercising, 88
mustard, 41
My Big Italian Veggie Bake (recipe), 174

N
napping, 112
90/10 rule, 4, 5
No-Oil Lemon Dressing (recipe), 191
nutritional supplements, 97–104
CBD (cannabidiol), 4, 100, 145–153
expiration date, 103
pro/prebiotics, 101–102
recommended supplements, 99–101
sleep-related supplements, 103
nuts and seeds, 27, 32, 54, 69, 70

O
oils
"good" oils, 28, 35, 55, 69
inflammation and, 35
oils to eliminate, 32, 35
partially hydrogenated oils, 35
One-Pan Chicken and Veggies (recipe), 210
One-Pan Chicken, Broccolini, and Squash (recipe), 214
One-Pot Shrimp Stew (recipe), 219
Overnight Chia Pudding (recipe), 193

P
pain
CBD (cannabidiol) and, 145, 147
exercise and, 87
pancakes, recipe, 197
pasta, 26, 67, 68
pectin, 102
phytonutrients, 51
pilaf, recipe, 182
Piña Colada Water (recipe), 229

ABOUT THE AUTHOR

Dr. Michael Rafael Moreno, better known as Dr. Mike, is a graduate of the University of California at Irvine and Hahnemann Medical School (now Drexel University). Following his internship and residency at Kaiser Permanente in Fontana, California, Dr. Mike moved to San Diego, where he currently practices family medicine, and served as physician lead for patient education and health promotion for a large medical group.

Since Dr. Mike Moreno first wrote *The 17 Day Diet* in 2010, millions of people have lost weight using his fast, safe, and extremely effective plan. Dr. Mike listens to his 17 Day dieters just as carefully as he listens to his own patients, and he is always on top of the cutting-edge research in the field of weight management. *The 17 Day Kickstart Diet* builds on the strong foundation he laid with *The 17 Day Diet*, by bringing in the most up-to-date information in the realms of nutrition, exercise, stress management, and supplementation.

Dr. Mike believes in creating programs that real people can follow in the real world. Life happens, and he wants to give his readers and patients the power to remain healthy, even when life gets complicated. As someone who doesn't just talk the talk, but who walks the walk, Dr.

Mike says, "I incorporate healthy habits into my work and home life, and you can too."

He is the author of *The 17 Day Diet*, *The 17 Day Diet Workbook*, *The 17 Day Diet Breakthrough Edition*, *The 17 Day Diet Cookbook*, and *The 17 Day Plan to Stop Aging*, as well as the host of the podcast *Wellness, Inc.*, which can be found on any of the major podcast platforms.